1996

THE FOR-PROFIT HEALTHCARE REVOLUTION

The Growing Impact of Investor-Owned Health Systems in America

THE FOR-PROFIT HEALTHCARE REVOLUTION
The Growing Impact of Investor-Owned Health Systems in America

Sandy Lutz and E. Preston Gee

A Healthcare 2000 Publication

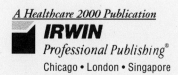

IRWIN
Professional Publishing®
Chicago • London • Singapore

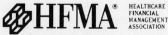

HEALTHCARE
FINANCIAL
MANAGEMENT
ASSOCIATION

A Healthcare 2000 Publication

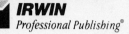

IRWIN
Professional Publishing®

© Richard D. Irwin, a Times Mirror Higher Education Group, Inc., company, 1995

Irwin Professional Book Team

Senior sponsoring editor: *Kristine Rynne*
Marketing manager: *Marissa Ramos*
Manager, direct marketing: *Rebecca S. Gordon*
Project editor: *Christina Thornton-Villagomez*
Production supervisor: *Lara Feinberg*
Assistant manager, desktop services: *Jon Christopher*
Designer: *Larry J. Cope*
Compositor: *David Corona Design*
Typeface: *11/13 Palatino*
Printer: *Buxton-Skinner Printing Co.*

▼▼ Times Mirror
M Higher Education Group

Library of Congress Cataloging-in-Publication Data

Lutz, Sandy
    The for-profit healthcare revolution : the growing impact of
investor-owned health systems in America / Sandy Lutz, E. Preston Gee.
      p.   cm.
    "A Healthcare 2000 publication
    Includes index.
    ISBN 1–55738–650–1
    1. Hospitals, Proprietary—United States. 2. Medical
corporations—United States.. I. Gee, Erin Preston. II. Title.
RA975.P74G44   1996
362.1'10973—dc20   95–23203
                                                CIP

Printed in the United States of America
 3 4 5 6 7 8 9 0

Contents

Foreword

The *For Profit Healthcare Revolution* is about a story that is still being written. If anything, the market forces which served as the crucible from which publicly owned community hospitals emerged have intensified. Cost pressures have never been greater. Competition has never been more fierce.

In some ways, it is difficult to comment on a story in which you are a character. But from another perspective, being a participant gives you a better appreciation for the challenges that faced the story's authors.

In chronicling the origins and growth of publicly held community hospitals and analyzing the market forces and business decisions that shaped this new industry, authors Sandy Lutz and E. Preston Gee have done a great service for consumers and purchasers of healthcare. By putting the past into perspective, they have assisted us in forecasting and preparing for a future that promises to bring even more sweeping change to healthcare.

Traditional concepts concerning who, how, and where healthcare is provided are being replaced with innovation upon innovation, driven by the recognition that the unbridled escalation of healthcare costs of the past can no longer be tolerated. Coupled with the mandate of controlling costs is the absolute necessity of maintaining and improving the quality of care that has become synonymous with our nation's healthcare system.

In many ways, the challenges faced by the hospital industry today are analogous to those of our nation's banking industry. Just as technological advances and economic pressures are causing banks to consolidate to form regional and national financial networks in which efficiency is gained while maintaining the convenience and product line demanded by an ever more sophisticated public, so too, the days of the stand-alone hospital are rapidly coming to a close.

A late 1995 study by the Pew Charitable Trust concluded that as many as half the nation's hospitals should probably be closed in the next decade and that the number of doctors, nurses and pharmacists be cut in half. As this is being written, the Congress of the United States is proposing to reduce Medicare and Medicaid spending by $450 billion over the next seven years. These are changes of cataclysmic proportions.

Columbia/HCA Healthcare Corporation was created with the belief that these massive changes would require a new model of patient care in which comprehensive, integrated patient care delivery networks would provide one source for patient care needs on the community, state and even national level. Sufficient size to create economies of scale and sufficient buying power to control supply costs were also part of the vision on which the company was built. Our efforts to build that company play a significant role in the story that unfolds in this book.

But at the heart of the Columbia vision was and is the belief that free-market, competitive forces should be the driver to bring about the change necessary to meet the healthcare challenges of the future. And the publicly held community hospital arena, in which competition breeds quality, efficiency, and choice, is the best medium to allow those forces to mold successful companies that can meet the expectations of individual consumers and large group purchasers of healthcare alike.

There are those who decry for-profit healthcare as something sinister or onerous, that healthcare is a basic human right that should not have a profit motive behind it. But just as competition forces the for-profit grocer to bring a greater variety of food at a better price, and the for-profit builder to create better and more affordable shelter, so too, the for-profit provider of healthcare is driven to increase quality and control costs to attract the consumer who generates the profits. No one would argue that food and shelter are less basic to a full life than healthcare, and no one argues the right and wrong of for-profit grocers and home builders. It should be no different with healthcare.

Consumers, employers and healthcare professionals themselves need to better understand the forces at work in the healthcare marketplace today and the future they are forging. This book is a great aid in moving forward that understanding.

This country is at a great crossroads in terms of how healthcare will be delivered to the American public in the future. New technology brings great promise. New models of healthcare delivery and management offer a chance to control costs. Innovative companies are forging new directions and partnerships to offer convenience and choice to the healthcare consumer. In tracing the evolution of healthcare and the impact of market forces upon it, authors Lutz and Gee have made a significant contribution to our understanding of what healthcare has become and provide assistance in preparing for what is yet to be.

In healthcare we have seen great change. Without a doubt, the change we've yet to see will be even greater. But as we strive to make those changes, we must never lose sight of the fact that in the final analysis, healthcare is and always must be extending a caring, healing hand to those in need. Whatever the delivery model, whatever the technology employed, the patient must come first. The healthcare company that wishes to be successful in the truest sense must keep that first and foremost in all it does. In the for-profit world of healthcare, seeing patients restored to their maximum ability to enjoy life is the ultimate bottom line.

Richard L. Scott
President/CEO, Columbia/HCA Healthcare Corporation

Introduction

What is the future of healthcare and who are the players that are shaping it? We believe you'll find some answers to these questions in the pages that follow.

This book reviews the genesis of the for-profit sector, the rationale for its creation, the factors leading to its days of decline, and its recent resurgence—or more descriptively, its recent revolution. Through a better understanding of the history of the players and firms that comprise the investor-owned market, we gain a better understanding of its current expansion, influence, and most importantly, its potential for the future.

Unlike some consumer-oriented industries, little has been written about the business executives who work in healthcare. As such, little is known about how financial and quality decisions are made in hospitals. Only in recent years have we heard talk about "report cards" on providers, but this discussion has centered more on health maintenance organizations than on hospitals and physicians specifically.

Medicine is a trillion-dollar business that embraces immense contradictions. The healthcare industry has evolved (and continues to do so) from an era where leaders were collegial to where they, by the very nature of the market, must be competitive. Healthcare providers are expected to be both charity-givers and profit-makers, compassioned servants and pragmatic entrepreneurs. A debate rages in the halls of medicine over which species is better for the hospital industry: investor-owned companies like the ones we describe in this book, or not-for-profit organizations that own the majority of this nation's hospitals.

We did not write this book to solve that debate. Instead, this book was conceived to shed light on the one species that—right or wrong—seems to be slowly winning the medical industry's evolutionary struggle. No other business is quite as complex as private medicine, and because of this, many important questions are never even asked much less answered. This book opens a window—albeit a small one—to that world. By focusing on the entrepreneurs who have carved a niche in the trillion-dollar business of healthcare, we are able to get a better understanding of the past, present, and future of perhaps the most important industry in America today.

One of the most prominent of these entrepreneurs is Rick Scott, sometimes referred to as "the Michael Jordan of healthcare." Whether or not you agree with this moniker, you cannot deny the influence his company, Columbia/HCA Healthcare Corporation, is having on the industry. Columbia/HCA and other for-profit companies are casting a large shadow throughout the industry, and their influence on the direction of healthcare simply cannot be ignored. While this book is not solely about Columbia, much of the text, especially the contemporary component, focuses on this rising giant. However, since Columbia is an amalgam of several of the original for-profit firms, the history and chronology of all the tax-paying players is highly relevant.

The first two chapters of this book deal with the history and early philosophy of the founding fathers and firms of the for-profit sector. This section is designed to give a synthesized review of these prominent players.

Chapter 3 offers a segue from the past—albeit relatively recent past—to the present, discussing the rationale for the current momentum and market-led changes affecting the industry. This discussion leads into our presentation and discussion of the contemporary companies with noted emphasis on Columbia/HCA. This latter review is contained in Chapters 4 and 5.

Chapter 6 is somewhat of a sidebar (nonetheless salient) that discusses the role of financing under the for-profit modus operandi. This section is especially relevant for observers of the industry concerned with either investing their own funds, or the collective investment involved in considering an organization's alignment with a tax-paying system.

Chapter 7 follows this tax-paying review with other considerations that boards and hospital executives should review in assessing their hospital's position vis à vis the for-profit entities—either as competitors or as allies. The final chapter offers the authors' (as well as pundits' and professionals') outlook on the future of the tax-paying sector and how that future will influence the industry.

OF PARAGRAPHS AND PROVISOS

As we conducted the research and began writing the text, we realized that the subject of the book did not have an agreed upon name. Consequently, you will read references like "investor owned," "for-profit," "tax-paying," and "proprietary," just to name a few. We recognize that some of these monikers will not please a few of our readers, but all of these synonyms are used in referencing the sector of the industry about which this book is based.

Rick Scott has been particularly vocal about the words "for-profit" being a misnomer since "not-for-profit" hospitals are often as profitable as "for-profit" ones. However, as we told him individually (when he voiced mild objection about the title of the book), the reality is that "for-profit" is the most common lexicon by which this sector of the industry is known.

Many of the executives that lead the charge today prefer the term "tax-paying" for their segment of the industry. However, this is a relatively recent appellation, and not without its own controversy. Many of the not-for-profit leaders dislike tax-referenced terminology (and the concomitant reference to their facilities as "tax-exempt"). Nonetheless, we use both terms frequently throughout the book.

Finally, it is not our intent to unnecessarily unnerve anyone in the process of reviewing the impact of the investor-owned sector. For better or worse, the nature of the healthcare industry has changed. What was once a cooperative environment has—for lack of a better term—"evolved" to a competitive one. Some view this as anathema to the very nature of healthcare. Perhaps this is true, but the current competitive environment would seem a reality against which historical idealism is ultimately doomed to fail.

This book is designed to provide all parties with a better perspective on the nature of a very significant force in a rapidly changing industry—namely the investor-owned companies and the individuals who lead them. To that extent, we hope the book achieves its objective.

Chapter 1

The For-Profit Founders and Firms

Shakespeare told us the past is prologue. Today's corporate hospital titans are testament to that, building their empires on foundations created by the men and women who created an investor-owned hospital industry in the 1960s. Some 1,300 hospitals today are investor-owned hospitals, meaning that they are owned by companies or individuals who answer to shareholders or other investors. These companies, which own about 20 percent of the nation's hospitals and 15 percent of the nation's 1.2 million hospital beds, also pay taxes.

The rest of the nation's hospitals are tax-exempt. They are the Baptists, Methodists, Catholic, and County Memorial hospitals of America. Some were founded as far back as 125 years ago by communities, church groups, or government entities.

Hospitals are the hub of today's trillion-dollar healthcare industry. Outpatient services, home health care, and physician services spin off and around that hub, but hospitals take home the lion's share—40 cents of every healthcare dollar.

Oddly enough, other segments of the health care industry aren't dominated by not-for-profit organizations. Most nursing homes, home health care agencies, pharmaceutical companies, and physician groups are taxpaying, for-profit organizations. Not so with hospitals.

While the differences between "for-profit" and "not-for-profit" hospitals used to be clear-cut, they are becoming less so. Critics of investor-owned systems charge that they revere profits to the detriment of quality patient care. Critics of tax-exempt systems say those hospitals don't provide enough charity care and community service to deserve their exemptions.

Arguably, in recent years, not-for-profit hospitals have started acting more like for-profit ones, adopting some of their business-school efficiencies and management techniques. Meanwhile, investor-owned hospitals have taken on some of the qualities of tax-exempt institutions, providing charity care and community service. In some cases, they have no choice. By federal law, no hospital—whether it be owned by the community or stockholders—can turn away emergency patients regardless of their ability to pay. What about nonemergency patients? In some small towns, the only hospital is an investor-owned one, making it hard to avoid giving away medical care to a patient who can't pay.

In the near future, "it will be difficult to tell the not-for-profits and the investor-owned hospitals apart," predicts Robert O'Leary, former president of one of the nation's largest investor-owned chains (American Medical International) and prior to that, of the largest not-for-profit hospital alliance (VHA). O'Leary now heads American Healthcare Systems, a San Diego-based alliance of 40 tax-exempt hospital systems.

He believes not-for-profit hospital systems will begin accessing the equity market. The alliance he now manages has a venture capital arm that invests in emerging technologies. Investor-owned chains, O'Leary believes, will see value in responding to a community's entire health needs. He maintains that they will focus on "providing care and treat profits as a derivative."

GOVERNMENT-PROMPTED REFORM

President Clinton tried to revolutionize the health care system in 1994, but his plan didn't get far in Congress. Nonetheless, the revolution did occur. His blueprint that fostered purchasing alliances inspired hundreds of hospitals to look for partners. If hospitals were forced to negotiate with large purchasing alliances, they needed to combine their clout. The desire to merge or be acquired reached its zenith in 1994 when over 650 hospitals—more than 10 percent of all U.S. hospitals—were caught up in merger and acquisition deals.

The Clinton plan wasn't the only impetus, though. If the Clinton plan was the spark, for-profit companies were the gasoline. Even when deals didn't involve them, the threat of Columbia/HCA Healthcare Corporation, or another investor-owned chain coming into their markets forced hospital boards into action.

The result? Like shares of IBM or futures in cotton, hospitals are now a commodity controlled by larger and larger corporations. Hospital corporations were born in the 1960s, then went through a retrenchment and restructuring period in the mid 1980s after Medicare introduced a new prospective payment system. Then, during the early 1990s, they entered a period of resurgence.

In each case, the nation's economy and government policy played a role in how these companies have fared. Is what's happening now just another reconfiguration? Will the pieces that stacked together to build Columbia into the nation's largest health care provider collapse into a heap of different shapes soon? In spite of the industry's rise and fall and rise again, a small circle of survivors seem to hang in there.

"There have been four different periods since 1968 that people said, 'Boy, you'd better get out of the hospital business. You're in trouble,'" said Thomas Frist Jr., M.D., who founded Hospital Corporation of America (HCA) and became chairman of Columbia when HCA merged with that organization in 1994.

Despite the warnings, the Nashville surgeon-turned-businessman didn't get out. In fact, he found that adversity created opportunity. That was true in 1994—one of the industry's most uncertain years because of Clinton's much ballyhooed promise to reform the nation's health care system. Yet, while health reform crashed and burned in the nation's capital, investor-owned chains were aggressively buying hospitals. Even tax-exempt systems were eyeing competitors to buy.

More than any other year, 1994 altered the fabric of the health care business in America's cities and towns. During that year, investor-owned chains, most notably Columbia, developed a disturbing predilection to "covet thy neighbor's hospital." That didn't necessarily set well with many in the not-for-profit dominated industry who cherished the collegial relationships of the past.

Witness this lead from a news article in the *Orlando Sentinel* dated March 25, 1995: "A document released Friday by a federal magistrate in Orlando appears to show a national hospital chain [Columbia] plotting to upset the balance of power among the region's largest hospitals." Plotting to upset the balance of power among the region's largest hospitals? Despicable. It causes one to wonder what horrible thing Columbia will do next.

Here is another extract, from the *San Diego Union*, March 16, 1995: "The nation's largest for-profit hospital chain [again, Columbia] has set its sights on buying control of hospitals and physician groups here, which could radically alter a regional marketplace dominated by non-profit, community hospitals."

As the adage goes, The meek may inherit the earth, but they'll never gain much market share. Investor-owned companies—such as Columbia—have long been bad mouthed, and often ignored, by the not-for-profit hospital sector. Purportedly, they skim the cream by treating only affluent patients, turn away the indigent, and drive up costs—or so the critics say.

In the past 20 years, some things have not changed. For-profit hospitals still get their share of bad-mouthing. However, they are no longer ignored. When a few men started for-profit hospital companies in the late 1960s, the thought of turning a profit on health care was considered an anathema by those on the "respectable"—the not-for-profit—side. After all, the traditionalists argued, people's lives are at stake in these institutions; profits shouldn't be a motivation.

In fact, some local hospital associations blackballed for-profit hospitals as late as the 1980s. A turning point came, however, when David Jones yanked the $333,000 membership of his Humana hospitals from the American Hospital Association (AHA) in December 1985. Humana, a Louisville, Kentucky-grown hospital chain, was a mighty power at the time.

Jones, its founder, (and a former Golden Gloves boxer), believed his company wasn't getting its money's worth from the AHA. Why fake a punch when you can jab? For not-for-profit executives, Jones' move was a wake-up call. Not only could for-profit chains threaten to use their economic clout, to weaken national associations, they would also follow through on their threats.

In the end, the not-for-profit hospitals that dominated the AHA succumbed to giving membership discounts to investor-owned chains of hospitals. Humana rejoined. Today, for-profit executives filter through state and national hospital groups, participating fully. It's hard to imagine these leaders not being included.

THOSE WHO FAIL TO LEARN THE LESSONS OF HISTORY . . .

Only the moment seems to exist. Individuals and hospitals get pushed down like a cork in the water, then later bob to the surface again. Different place, different circumstances. As the saying goes, you can't keep a good man (or even a scoundrel, for that matter) down.

Since the industry's growth isn't well chronicled, is it doomed to repeat the mistakes of the past? When asked what today's generation of hospital companies learned from the previous generation, a CEO of a top hospital chain answered, "Zero." He went on to say that, "In the past, the span of control of hospitals has been about 100 hospitals. When they run over 100, they get into trouble."

Such an observation is especially chilling considering that one company, Columbia/HCA Healthcare Corp., has swallowed more than one-third of the investor-owned industry following its latest deal, the $5.6 billion acquisition of Healthtrust in 1995. In other words, one company practically dominates a movement that has been a battering ram in one of the nation's largest industries.

Is Columbia—now the nation's 10th largest employer—a General Motors for the health care industry? Just as three automotive companies dominate the domestic car industry, will Columbia and a few other health care companies direct the future of this trillion-dollar sector?

If the past is indeed prologue, Columbia will grow and grow. Then it will break up in a wave of divestitures and restructuring—that is, if the brief history of privately owned health care companies were to repeat itself. Columbia executives say that would never happen; their company (which during 1994, according to *Fortune Magazine*, was the nation's 14th fastest growing corporation) is different. Yet, looking at investor-owned chains of the past, it's wise to never say never, or perhaps, never say forever.

Perhaps the best illustration of this dynamic comes from considering the list of publicly held hospital companies in 1984. The ensuing financial and organizational chaos make a decade seem like a lifetime in the world of investor-owned chains.

- American Medical International—acquired in 1995 by National Medical Enterprises, which changed its name to Tenet Healthcare Corp.

- Basic American Medical—purchased by Columbia Hospital Corp. (which later became Columbia/HCA) in 1992.
- Charter Medical Corp.—still around, but hobbled by debt from a leveraged buyout and payers' refusal to fund long lengths of stay in psychiatric hospitals.
- Community Psychiatric Centers—battered by the slump in the industry and transforming itself into a subacute hospital company, an industry sector that pays better than psychiatric care.
- Comprehensive Care Corp.—nearly exited the hospital business, another casualty of payers' perception that psychiatric hospitals were running up their charges in the late 1980s.
- HEI Corp.—bought by Columbia in 1990.
- Hospital Corp. of America—bought by Columbia in 1994.
- Humana—broke into two parts in 1993, an insurance company and a hospital company. Its hospitals, under the new name of Galen Health Care, were bought by Columbia in 1993.
- National Medical Enterprises—hit bottom in 1994 with restructuring, lawsuits, federal criminal investigations, and financial problems, but could emerge as one of the major players. Acquired AMI in 1995 and changed its name to Tenet Healthcare Corporation.
- Nu-Med—Recently emerged from bankruptcy reorganization.
- Republic Health Corp.—Now called OrNda, the company went through a bankruptcy reorganization, changed its name, its management, and its address.
- Summit Health—bought by OrNda in 1994.
- Universal Health Services—Still around, although the chain recently bought and sold a handful of hospitals.

So, of the above-listed companies, four were bought by Columbia, three went through bankruptcy reorganization, three merged with each other, and another four have had severe financial problems stemming from their psychiatric operations. Even more noteworthy is the fact that only one, Universal, remains in its current form with the same top management.

This synoptic review of the founding firms underscores a critical issue that we will discuss throughout this book: How many boards of trustees consider this historical context when selling a hospital that's been owned by a community for decades? As mentioned earlier, the history of privately held hospital firms is either too brief or too inchoate to have merited the type of review and documentation one would expect (and hope for) from such a powerful sector of the industry. The analytical review is also disappointingly sparse when considered from the standpoint of individuals who must make strategic decisions about their institutions. These decisions— regarding alignment with taxpaying companies—have long-term implications, but are inherently based on short-term experience. This is one of the most perplexing dilemmas facing health industry leaders, who continually query, "What is this Columbia organization all about?"

This latter dilemma is analogous to the literary critic who commented on the autobiography of a 30-something luminary, "I never give much credence to a biography about anyone under 40, because they haven't lived long enough, nor done enough, to tell you much about their true self." Those health care executives who want to determine the true nature of Columbia (and some of the other taxpaying health care firms) face a similar fate: trying to predict the future status and professional character of a nascent firm.

The fits and starts of America's for-profit hospital companies have not been an exercise in futility, however. They've altered this industry and the way it competes. History shows that there have been plenty of mistakes, as well as examples of bad timing and considerable ambition—bordering on greed.

Perhaps the best example of such behavior was provided by National Medical Enterprises (NME) and its psychiatric hospitals. Under tremendous pressure to fill beds in the late 1980s, NME executives and professionals in the psychiatric hospitals purportedly paid doctors, school counselors, and other mental health workers to refer patients to them.

One of NME's founders, John Bedrosian, had license plates that read ADC, which stood for average daily census. The acronym on the license plate symbolized the focus of the firm. Administrators and others were judged (and compensated) on how many beds were full, or in hospital parlance, the census of the hospital.

What goes around comes around, though, and NME eventually paid for its questionable ethics when it was fined a record $379 million by the federal government in 1994 after a wide-ranging fraud investigation.

However, NME's founders started with good intentions. "One of the joys I used to have in this business when we started the business was to know that we thought we were doing something that had a social good attached to it," Bedrosian said in a deposition taken in connection with NME's patient fraud lawsuits.

Despite these publicized transgressions, the investor-owned industry glistens with examples of courage and vision as well. Certainly that was the case with Humana and Hospital Corp. of America, which pushed the boundaries of hospital operations into new frontiers. Both companies rose to prominence, taking on new challenges that eventually proved to be too soon, too grand, and perhaps, even too self-serving.

After all, this is a heady business. Even the smallest hospital chain amounts to a multimillion-dollar business. Even the smallest hospital deals in human lives. Put that on a grand scale, and one realizes that this industry cannot be compared to any other.

Not only is health care one of the nation's biggest businesses, it's also one of the most prestigious. The world beats a path to our hospitals. Humana founder David Jones used to say, "Get me an American who's sick in Germany and the first words out of his mouth are going to be, 'I want to go home.'"

It's no coincidence that Humana—after it had been emulated for its financial skills—aimed to become a world leader in medicine with the artificial heart transplants in 1984. It could have been the company's zenith. Instead, it began a series of missteps that   led to Humana's multimillion-dollar losses and the company's dismantling.

Still, Humana's David Jones and HCA's Thomas Frist Jr., M.D. have been hailed as visionaries. Unfortunately, vision sometimes clashes with reality for companies whose fate is in the hands of the stock market. When growth is dictated by shareholder value—getting a higher price for the company's stock—vision may be compromised by the discipline required to produce quarterly earnings gains.

Once a company is owned by shareholders, it puts certain financial formulas into motion: return on equity, return on investment, price/earnings ratios. The wheels start cranking on a moving sidewalk toward bigger and bigger profits. Stop the sidewalk and stockholders will abandon you in droves.

IN THE BEGINNING, THERE WAS MEDICARE . . .

What put the sidewalk's gears into motion in the first place? Arguably, it was Medicare. Introduced as part of President Lyndon Johnson's own vision of a great society, Medicare paid hospitals and physicians to treat the elderly. Medicare was one of many taxpayer-supported programs developed by the Johnson administration that made Americans more dependent on government.

In the case of health care, Medicare became the single largest customer for doctors and hospitals. It proved to be a great arrangement for hospitals. Essentially, the federal government gave hospitals a blank check: Just add up your costs, fill in the blank and Uncle Sam will reimburse you. The more you spend, the more you get paid.

"You couldn't lose money," said Nashville businessman Joel Gordon of those palmy days of Medicare. A cash flow spigot was turned on and hospital use by Americans over age 65 quadrupled within four years of the program's introduction. The country suddenly needed more and more hospitals. Gordon started a nursing home company, General Care Corporation, in 1969 in Nashville, but quickly switched to hospitals when a group of doctors urged him to convert a 250-bed nursing home into one.

Gordon realized the idea was sound, and soon he and his team traveled the countryside, meeting with doctors who wanted to build hospitals. General Care would hold a 51 percent interest in the new hospital; the doctors would take 49 percent.

On the West Coast, Uranus "Bob" Appel formed American Medical International from a laboratory company he started in 1956. A microbiologist by training, he bought his first two hospitals in 1960 and raised a whopping $180,000 in the company's initial public offering.

Up until the 1960s, the hospitals primarily were owned by churches, like the Catholics, Methodists, and Baptists. Some doctors owned hospitals as well, but there were no hospital companies; chains were organizations for fast-food restaurants and department stores, not hospitals.

When the Federation of American Hospitals—a splinter group that represents only for-profit hospitals—formed in 1966, nearly all of its members were doctors. Yet, others were seeing the financial potential provided by Medicare, and corporate chains began popping up here and there. The industry's tax-exempt majority didn't appreciate these interlopers, though.

THE INVESTOR-OWNED SECTOR IS BORN

A hospital developer from Portland, Oregon, Eugene Brim, was one of the Federation's founders who grappled with ill will from tax-exempt hospitals. "There was such antagonism from not-for-profits who labeled the corporate hospital owners as 'proprietary,'" said Brim.

Brim and others didn't like that name. At an early meeting of Federation members, "I said, 'what about investor-owned?'" Brim recalled. With that, a moniker was born. In 1969, Michael Bromberg was hired as the Federation's executive director and the complexion of the organization, now called the Federation of American Health Care Systems, started to change. "I remember our board switched overnight almost from doctors to businessmen," Bromberg said.

By 1970, several chains had formed—American Medical International (the first for-profit hospital chain), National Medical Enterprises, Hospital Corp. of America, and Humana.

HCA—THE PROPRIETARY PATRIARCH

Tommy Frist Jr. was a 28-year-old Air Force flight surgeon with time on his hands to think while stationed in Georgia during the early 1960s. He knew of Kemmons Wilson, who started a chain of hotels called Holiday Inns. The young doctor began to think of the 5,000 hospitals in America and how they might be similarly linked.

"I just plagiarized the concept," he explained. He returned to Nashville and talked to his dad, Thomas Frist Sr., who coincidentally needed to find a buyer for Park View Hospital, a Nashville, hospital that he had helped found in 1960. Father and son linked up with two other key men: the late Jack Massey, who created a $500 million empire known as Kentucky Fried Chicken (KFC) and Henry Hooker, a founder of the lesser-known enterprise, Minnie Pearl's Chicken. Together, they started the company, in which each of the four held equal shares.

Six months later, Hooker dropped out, but Massey was in for good. Three years after founding Hospital Corporation of America (HCA) with Frist, Massey, who was credited with creating the fast-food industry, resigned as KFC's chairman to concentrate on a new horizon as chairman of HCA. In a May 30, 1970, article in *Business Week*, Massey said that selling fried chicken and running hospitals had a lot in common: "The secret is in the management."

Not-for-profit hospital executives scoffed at these upstarts. Calling Massey and HCA "chicken pluckers," John R. Gadd, a director of Lee Memorial Hospital in Fort Myers, Florida, told *Business Week* that the for-profits were only providing the services with high profit margins, ignoring obstetrics and emergency rooms.

How irrelevant that argument seems today. With many investor-owned hospitals in the suburbs, obstetrics are a popular product line. As for emergency rooms, not many hospitals these days can get licensed without one.

Hospital Corp. of America went public in 1969, selling 400,000 shares. The stock was an instant hit. On the first day of trading, HCA stock jumped from $18 to $46 per share. Success breeds copycats. By 1971, there were 38 investor-owned hospital chains, more than a dozen of which were traded on the major stock exchanges.

The hospital corporate chains were starting to attract attention. An article in the November 1974 *Harvard Business Review* noted the criticism of investor-owned chains: "cream-skimmers" who take only the highest-paying patients. Similar charges (of skimming the cream) have been made against competitors in other regulated industries, such as the postal service and the telephone systems, the article pointed out. "The charge that profit-making hospitals are

less costly because they cut too many corners seems hard to rec-
oncile with another charge—that they cater only to affluent patients. Why would affluent patients settle for inadequate services?"
the article questioned.

During the next few years, HCA built hospitals. Most were in the
South, to which the population was migrating and cities didn't have
the money to build their own hospitals. Often, those cities didn't
want to turn to a for-profit company, but they didn't have any other
choice.

Many community hospitals had been built with funds through
the Hill-Burton Act, a 1946 initiative in which Congress adminis-
tered funds to build hospitals. By the 1960s, those funds had ebbed,
and hospital corporations such as HCA stepped in to finance the
South's new hospitals.

The government, in fact, was doing little to encourage the industry. In 1973, President Nixon proposed a broad health care cost
containment effort. The legislation that passed endorsed a new
concept called health maintenance organizations (HMOs). The new
product didn't exactly capture consumers' fancy. Notably, after 20
years, HMOs are emerging as a dominant player in the health care
industry.

Government policy continued to make the industry's future look
dim. In 1977, Health Education and Welfare (HEW) Secretary Joseph Califano proposed decertifying 100,000 inpatient beds so that
hospitals had to maintain a minimum 85 percent occupancy rate.
President Carter proposed the Hospital Cost Containment Act of
1977, calling for a 9 percent cap on hospital revenue increases. Wall
Street worried whether such measures might hinder the revenue
growth of hospital chains. (By the way, a one-day hospital stay in
1977 cost $158).

On the economic front, interest rates were brimming and would
hit 16 percent by 1979.

HCA GOES ON THE ACQUISITION TRAIL

Fortunately for the industry, the administration's proposals went
nowhere, and soon Frist was on the acquisition trail.

Massey had set a goal of having 100 hospitals in 10 years, and he was determined to meet it. In 1978, he recruited Donald MacNaughton, who had been Prudential Insurance Corporation's CEO since 1969. He was one of America's most recognized CEOs, but at the age of 61 had decided to pass the post on to the next guy and look for another job.

Massey called, thinking MacNaughton would give the younger Frist and his colleagues some seasoned management combined with large corporate experience. After all, MacNaughton had traded managing Prudential's $46 billion in assets for HCA's much smaller $707 million.

In 1980, HCA bought Gordon's General Care, a 12-hospital chain, for $78 million and then followed in 1981 with the acquisition of Hospital Affiliates, HCA's hometown competitor, for $950 million. A Nashville, Tennessee-based firm that owned or leased 57 hospitals and managed another 102 facilities, Hospital Affiliates jump-started HCA's climb to the top.

Good timing was a cornerstone of the Hospital Affiliates deal. At a March 25, 1981, board meeting, INA, a Philadelphia-based insurer, had already decided to sell Affiliates. Two days later, MacNaughton called and offered to buy it, not knowing that INA had decided to sell.

Within weeks, the deal was done.

MacNaughton's good fortune in snagging Affiliates also indirectly jump-started a health care economic development boom in Nashville as several executives from Hospital Affiliates went on to start their own companies. Just as Federal Express recharged Memphis, and General Motors built Detroit, HCA created an industry for Nashville beyond the wailing steel guitars of country music.

HCA built fortunes for its executives and their families; it nurtured entrepreneurs who would start some 20 publicly held health care companies, including PhyCor, Allied Clinical Labs, Hospital Management Professionals, and Coventry Corp. All of this health care spawning and subdividing occurred alongside not-for-profit powerhouses such as Baptist and St. Thomas hospitals in a city of a half million residents.

Investor-owned health care executives created their own clique that played by different tax rules. PhyCor, for example, was formed by 10-year HCA veteran Joseph Hutts. PhyCor actually created another investor-owned health care industry that is blossoming: ownership and management of physician groups.

Hospital Affiliates executives formed two other hospital chains: Republic Health Corporation, which went through a series of financial restructuring before emerging as OrNda HealthCorp., and Community Health Systems, a Houston-based hospital chain that found success managing rural and suburban hospitals. Another spawn was Medical Care America, a Dallas-based firm, led by former Affiliates executive Don Steen and purchased by Columbia for $860 million in 1994.

Nashville became a laboratory for health care companies whose executives had learned the ropes at HCA. It was like having a corporate mentor as a neighbor. Financing was there too. Third National Bank funded HCA, Hospital Affiliates, and General Care, in Nashville as well as Humana in Louisville. Third National's former chairman, Charles Kane, served on HCA's board and is now on Columbia's as well. Those companies "offered an opportunity to add a little more business management to the health care industry," Kane said. Massey's company, Masssey Burch Investment Group, still operates in Nashville, providing venture capital funding to young health care companies.

HCA "served as a model to people who had entrepreneurial spirit." "They'd say, 'They're no smarter than I am; I can do that too,'" said Surgical Care's Gordon. HCA helped Gordon finance an outpatient surgery center chain. With two million dollars from HCA and a six million dollar line of credit, Gordon formed Surgical Care Affiliates, today the largest independent surgery center chain.

In the 1980s, HCA was a builder with Tommy Frist, Jr. as its architect. By this time, Thomas Frist, Sr. had turned the reins over to his son. Although not-for-profits often discounted this "offshoot" of the industry, HCA was attracting talented executives who believed in the Frists' determination and ethics.

"They really ran the business like you were taught in Sunday School," said Stanton Tuttle, who joined HCA in 1980 and was one of its top three executives before leaving in 1986. "Whatever you told anybody verbally, you'd honor."

Executives didn't have written contracts because they knew Tommy Frist was good for his word. "They treated people right," Tuttle said.

HCA PURSUES A NOT-FOR-PROFIT

By the early 1980s, Frist was getting good feedback about his investor-owned company. "We had proven we could be responsible corporate citizens," he said. It was time for some big moves. Those moves soon came knocking at the door of not-for-profit health care. Frist initiated a move that became a disturbing wake-up call to his tax-exempt competitors. It was akin to David Letterman moving from NBC to CBS or Wayne Gretsky leaving Canada to play hockey for a U.S. team.

The board of Wesley Medical Center, a 760-bed teaching hospital in Wichita, Kansas, agreed to sell the not-for-profit hospital to HCA for $265 million in late 1984. The buyout stunned administrators at not-for-profit hospitals, especially those who belonged to Voluntary Hospitals of America (VHA), a growing not-for-profit alliance that Wesley's former CEO, Roy House, helped found.

Just three years earlier, VHA's new CEO Don Arnwine had been featured on the cover of *Modern Healthcare* with the headline: "VHA: Can volunteerism stop the investor-owned companies?" Not-for-profit hospitals hoped so. They were buying shares in the alliance and combining their purchasing clout to get vendor discounts on everything from intravenous pumps to surgical supplies.

After all, VHA's member CEOs ran large not-for-profit hospitals and wanted some of the same advantages as investor-owned chains. Clearly, VHA was designed to help hospitals such as Wesley compete with for-profits such as HCA. Now, here was Wesley caving in to the "enemy."

Unlike today, when many hospital CEOs follow a career ladder that sometimes bounces between investor-owned hospitals and not-for-profits, back in the early days of investor-owned chains, administrators only worked one side of the street. Predictably, investor-owned hospitals were considered adversaries. What's more, no one expected investor-owned chains to just waltz in and buy large, prestigious, not-for-profit medical centers. Trustees wouldn't make the time to listen to the sales pitch.

Instead, for-profits stuck to building their own hospitals or scooping up financially struggling institutions. Consequently, the Wesley sale was a bolt from the blue.

"It was one of the biggest 'whys' of my life," said Don Arnwine, the former VHA president, now a private consultant. Arnwine remembers the only answer he received came from the hospital's CEO, A.B. "Jack" Davis, who told Arnwine that he saw "storm clouds on the horizon." Congress was debating cutbacks in reimbursement, and utilization was forecast to drop—not unlike the dire predictions that circle the industry today. "In retrospect, the storm clouds people are seeing today are much, much darker," Arnwine said, adding, "It still remains a giant puzzle to me."

In those days, hospital acquisitions were typically valued on a dollar-per-bed calculation, and the Wesley buy was a staggering $348,684 per bed. Arnwine points out that even today, few institutions of Wesley's reputation have been scooped up by for-profit chains. In 1994, Columbia agreed to merge its Atlanta hospitals with Emory University, a highly regarded health care system. However, that deal eventually imploded, in part because Emory heard negative feedback from several smaller Georgia hospitals from which it received referrals.

The Wesley deal stirred passions. Roy House, who had been Wesley's CEO for 24 years before retiring in 1981, returned to Wichita to try to convince the board not to do the HCA deal. "Roy had spent virtually his entire career and was personally invested in that place in a way few people are today," Arnwine said. "He had taken it from a little 20-bed hospital to the preeminent institution in that part of the country."

Even so, the die was cast. Although some Methodist officials initially balked at the deal, they were assuaged by a reported $32 million from sale proceeds that would be used to fund a new foundation.

A trend was starting, and the Wesley announcement was followed by another blockbuster sale of a not-for-profit. In March 1985, Presbyterian-St. Luke's Medical Center in Denver agreed to be sold to American Medical International in Beverly Hills for $178 million. HCA also had bid for Presbyterian but lost out to AMI. Nonetheless, HCA gobbled up other large not-for-profits in Oklahoma, Utah, and New Mexico.

For example, in February 1985, HCA purchased 80 percent of Lovelace Medical Center, an Albuquerque, New Mexico, hospital that was among the best positioned facilities in the industry for the coming wave of managed care. Lovelace is a group practice clinic, like The Mayo Clinic in Rochester, Minnesota, or The Ochsner Foundation in New Orleans. The advantage of such structures lies in the incentive arrangement, under which both the hospital and the doctors are aligned in the same organization.

Amazingly, in less than one year, HCA had purchased more than $1 billion in tax-exempt hospitals. Frist recalled that many advisers told him not to buy teaching hospitals such as Wesley. "Those were some of the best decisions we ever made," he countered. "It took us to a new level." Critics who charged that HCA wasn't interested in teaching, research, and charity could only scratch their heads at HCA's new acquisitions. However, the biggest bombshell was still to come.

HCA AND AMERICAN HOSPITAL SUPPLY

On April Fool's Day 1985, HCA and American Hospital Supply Corporation (American) announced that they would merge into a vertically integrated healthcare company, an $8.5 billion corporation. Frist and American's CEO, the late Karl Bays, explained to a stunned industry that the merger was a way for both companies to save money and expand. A giant manufacturer and distributor of all kinds of hospital supplies, American could be folded into the HCA corporate structure, cutting a wide swath through HCA's purchasing costs.

Together, the merged companies—to be called Kuron—could borrow as much as one billion dollars to buy more hospitals, more HMOs, and more pharmaceutical manufacturers. Or so Frist and Bays reasoned.

By this time, HCA was a powerhouse, owning or managing 366 acute-care hospitals with 54,324 beds, 28 psychiatric hospitals with 3,619 beds, and 27 foreign hospitals with 2,722 beds. It also owned 17 percent of Beverly Enterprises, the nation's largest nursing home chain.

Because of its size, HCA was beginning to feel boxed in. Investor-owned chains were still located primarily in the South, and the company was risking antitrust problems if it expanded too much. Frist knew the company had to keep growing. The question was how? "I thought about putting together a GE (General Electric) of healthcare," he explained. "GE owns Kidder Peabody and other lines of business."

Yet, some of Frist's own men were telling him the merger with American could backfire. Not-for-profits were starting to hate HCA and they would surely not do anything that would fatten its coffers. Frist's executives knew this, warning him that American's other hospital customers would abandon the company once it became a part of HCA. Large purchasing groups of not-for-profit hospitals, such as VHA and the Daughters of Charity, the nation's largest Catholic hospital system, could pull as much as $500 million in American's business.

Despite the warnings from inside their own companies, Frist and Bays pressed ahead. HCA signed a five-year lease in a Nashville office building for the proposed company, Kuron, sure that the deal would go through. "There was so much underlying value," Frist explained. "I had an exit strategy."

Frist figured he could sell the distribution business or the manufacturing business off if things didn't work out. Bays himself was talking to Arnwine about Voluntary Hospitals of America buying the company's distribution business. VHA was an alliance of large not-for-profit hospitals that had started a purchasing program with Bays' help. Bays and Arnwine became personal friends, and Bays pleaded with Arnwine to keep the alliance's business.

Almost immediately after the announcement, both companies' worst fears were realized. VHA, Daughters of Charity, and Humana gave American 60 days notice. They were pulling their business.

Even worse, Wall Street revolted. HCA and American stocks both dropped more than $2.50 a share. "How would this deal fill hospital beds?" one Wall Street analyst questioned. Many saw the move merely as a grab for growth, and an ill-advised one at that. However, American's mate for life was waiting in the wings. Baxter Travenol, another Chicago-area hospital supply firm, swept in with a hostile offer. American rejected the offer, and an irate HCA canceled its $40 million intravenous supply contract with Baxter in retaliation for the hostile interference. HCA raised its offer, but Baxter upped its ante to 53 dollars a share, about one million dollars more than HCA was offering, for a total price of $3.6 billion.

Inexplicably, HCA folded its cards in retreat. With that, Bays' great vision melted away. "Bays said he felt like Tommy Frist left him in the middle of Lake Michigan without any oars," commented one source about HCA's decision not to outbid Baxter. Yet, Frist answers: "It only made sense to go down that path if you paid the right amount." In the end, Bays would become chairman of Baxter, but leave the health care industry 18 months later to head IC Industries, a Chicago-based conglomerate.

Actually, HCA emerged from the battle in strong financial shape. It withdrew its bid—taking a $150 million payoff for its trouble. What's more, HCA was promised another $50 million in 1991 if HCA bought more than $1.325 billion in supplies over the next five years.

HCA HEALTH PLANS: THE START OF A DOWNWARD SLIDE

HCA then decided to follow the lead of Humana, diving into the insurance business. With a bravado that was becoming characteristic, HCA announced that it was launching HCA Health Plans in the summer of 1985.

Company officials said they expected to have one million subscribers by December 1987 and insurance revenues of one billion dollars by 1988. The plan was for HCA to offer a host of health plans, not just an HMO. To get started, the chain bought a Los Angeles HMO with 16,000 members for $24 million. Company officials said they planned to spend another $125 million to buy other health plans in 1985.

For a while, the future looked rosy. A consultants' strategic report to top HCA executives in 1986 predicted that HCA would be an $11 billion company by 1992. It was not to be. In the second quarter, ending June 30, 1985, HCA reported a 26 percent drop in profits, to $67 million. Frist blamed a $7.2 million loss in its health plan business and said that hospital occupancy had dropped to 48 percent. Patient days were down 2.3 percent compared to the previous year.

Things didn't look as though they were going to get better soon. The Reagan administration had just proposed a thin, half-percent increase in Medicare rates for 1987. Almost the entire industry entered a slump. Republic Health Corporation—started by former Hospital Affiliates executives—mortgaged itself to the hilt with a management-led leveraged buyout (LBO) in the fall of 1986 and immediately hit a financial wall.

Republic had purchased 18 money-losing hospitals from HCA for $215 million and had managed to turn them around. However, the magic didn't last. The LBO was more than the company could bear. With more than $800 million in high-yield debt, Republic soon began gagging on its $25 million in quarterly interest payments. It was losing $2 million a week on operations and began to frantically search for buyers for its hospitals.

Trouble was, the now slumping industry was full of distressed properties. Republic's hospitals were only one-third full, and insiders soon realized the company's debt exceeded the value of its assets. Analysts valued Republic's hospitals at about $600 million. In other words, if you managed to find buyers for everything, you still couldn't pay off the debt. Republic wasn't the only hospital chain in trouble.

American Healthcare Management (AHM), another Dallas-based chain, began having cash flow troubles and was forced into Chapter 11 bankruptcy reorganization in the fall of 1987. Amid a vicious battle with its banks, the company finally reemerged from bankruptcy two years later.

American Healthcare's top executives, like many of their cohorts, blamed Medicare's new diagnosis-related groups (DRG) system—which paid hospitals a fixed amount based on a patient's diagnosis—rather than their own missteps. AHM's executives didn't survive the bankruptcy reorganization.

In 1987, only half of the nation's hospitals made a profit on patient operations, according to HCIA, a Baltimore research firm that specializes in hospital financial information. Medicare margins had been in the 14 percent range in 1984. As a result of DRGs, the margins dropped to 5 percent by 1987, according to the Health Care Financing Administration (HCFA), the government agency that oversees Medicare.

"A lot of the companies during the 80s argued that a lot of their problems were related to DRGs," said Steve Volla, who was brought in to turn around American Healthcare Management. After righting the ship at AHM, he engineered a merger with OrNda HealthCorp, a Nashville, Tennessee-based hospital chain in 1984. (Since then, Volla's gone on to start another hospital company, Primary Health Systems.) "Yet, DRGs in the 1980s were an easy scapegoat. It showed that some companies weren't ready," Volla now says, adding, "We're still with the same DRG system, and the for-profits still are handsomely surviving."

HCA PARES DOWN TO THE CORE

Size didn't necessarily insulate America's largest hospital chain, HCA. What happened to HCA is often viewed as an example of what could happen to today's Columbia. By 1987, HCA owned 225 U.S. hospitals and 25 foreign hospitals and had management contracts to operate another 200 hospitals. Still, Frist was forced to dismantle the empire in the name of shareholder value.

First, he streamlined costs, taking $125 million in annual corporate overhead and cutting it to $28 million. Then, the divestitures began. On August 31, 1987, he spun off 104 hospitals—widely regarded as "the marginal performers"—to Healthtrust in a $2.1 billion deal. Of course, HCA kept its jewel, Wesley in Wichita, a 760-bed lion with a strong 71 percent occupancy.

Although the Healthtrust spin-off positioned HCA as a stronger company, it didn't help the stock price. To boost shareholder value, HCA proposed buying back 12 million shares at $47 per share in September. Then came the October 1987 stock market crash, which hammered HCA shares down to $30.

To make matters worse, the financial windfall from selling hospitals to Healthtrust didn't look like such a great success on the books. Although HCA recorded a $300 million gain on the sale of Healthtrust, the SEC said it had to defer the profit to future periods. The result was that HCA was forced to pay taxes on the gain of $140 million. That resulted in a $58 million loss in 1987.

The stock buyback at $47 per share paid shareholders a premium, yet HCA stock continued to languish in the low- to mid-30s through much of 1988. Fearing a takeover of the family-started business, Frist (in September 1988) proposed a leveraged buyout to take HCA private at $51 per share. Going private would also take HCA—whose stability was the opposite extreme of other investor-owned hospital firms such as AMI—off the market for takeovers.

Interestingly, in 1987, Frist and his board had rebuffed an out-of-the-blue offer from two former Republic Health executives and their attorney Richard Scott. That incident would be the catalyst for

Scott's remarkable rise in the hospital industry. Several months later, Scott founded Columbia Hospital Corp. with Fort Worth, Texas, financial whiz Richard Rainwater.

"I didn't even know who he was," Frist said about Scott. "That's how ridiculous the era was. He had $25,000 in his pocket, and he was offering to buy a $5 billion company." Frist realized that if an unknown like Rick Scott could marshal enough junk bond capital to take over his company, he'd better do something.

Takeover fever had gripped Wall Street, which at the time was atwitter with the celebrated bidding war for RJR Nabisco. That $25-billion megadeal for the cigarette and cookie giant later spawned a book and movie, *Barbarians at the Gate*, about the "insanity" surrounding Wall Street's wheeler dealers.

HCA's deal—the largest leveraged buyout (LBO) in the history of the hospital industry—would appear small by comparison, but prove vastly more successful than the much ballyhooed RJR transaction. Kohlberg Kravis Roberts & Co., known as KKR, won the bidding in history's largest LBO ever.

KKR, considering a counteroffer for HCA, had looked at the company's books after Frist and his managers made a bid for the company. Intent on winning RJR, KKR partner Henry Kravis diverted his attention away from HCA. Ironically, RJR chairman Ross Johnson lost his company to KKR. Tommy Frist did not lose his firm.

Amid talks that Humana might make an offer, Frist and his managers ended up being the only bidders for HCA, which became a private company once again in March 1989. KKR's deal for RJR Nabisco closed within a week of HCA's. Frist saw Kravis a week after that.

The HCA founder congratulated the Wall Street baron for winning RJR, then asked him why he hadn't pursued HCA. "Tommy," Kravis said, "I understand Oreo cookies better than I do DRGs."

HCA's LBO burdened the hospital company with a staggering $4.5 billion in debt. However, none of it was high-yield junk bond debt. Frist himself pledged 100 percent of net worth, and 21 officers of HCA pledged half of their net worth to get the loans. The company was 90 percent leveraged and its debt was costing $85,000 an hour, Frist recalled.

Radical surgery had to be done to pare costs and sell assets so that HCA could begin to repay its debt. The company's contract management group was sold to senior managers and Welsh Carson Anderson & Stowe, a New York-based venture capital firm, for $44 million. Renamed Quorum Health Group and led by longtime HCA executive, James Dalton, Quroum emerged as a hospital chain in its own right.

Frist also sold the company's British and Australian hospitals and was poised to sell a highly valued asset: the psychiatric business. Over the preceding few years, HCA had built the nation's largest chain of freestanding psychiatric hospitals, with 6,000 beds. The psychiatric division had the highest operating margins in HCA and the fastest growth. While medical-surgical hospitals were struggling, the psychiatric facilities were going like gang busters.

The math worked out perfectly. The psychiatric hospitals would be sold for $1.6 billion. HCA could take the proceeds to repay a $1.3-billion bridge loan taken out to finance the LBO. Frist's idea was to sell the mental health business to its employees, the same way it had with Healthtrust. Employee stock ownership plans (ESOPs) were a hot trend. AMI had orchestrated a similar arrangement, selling its less profitable hospitals to an ESOP, Epic Healthcare Group, in 1988.

Nonetheless, the deal was a struggle from day one. Starting in March 1989, Jim Don, president of the psychiatric company, and Vic Campbell, HCA's vice president of investor relations, took the proposed arrangement to New York, visiting with high-level executives from Chase Manhattan, Bankers Trust, Citicorp, and Bank of Nova Scotia.

After the presentations, the bankers cornered Don. "What do you really think?" they asked. Don was in a precarious position. On one hand he was representing a new company that would have to pay off a $1-billion-plus loan. On the other hand, he was a long-time HCA executive, loyal to Frist and the company. "I was kind of caught in the middle," Don said later.

In the July 24, 1989, issue of *Forbes*, the questionable economics of the deal hit the fan. The article, headlined "A crazy deal?", charged that Frist was forcing his employees to pay "through the nose" for the psychiatric business. The magazine also suggested that the U.S. Labor Dept.—the watchdog of ESOPs—should look into HCA's proposal.

Weeks passed. The industry was changing quickly, and not for the better. Though few could have predicted it at the time, the psychiatric inpatient business was within a year of going into a deep and dangerous tailspin, motored by overbuilding and greed. The overbuilding would bring aggressive advertising campaigns and tactics that would turn the industry into a financial nightmare.

By late 1989, negative news stories began sprouting about the inappropriate hospitalization of teenagers. That, coupled with uncertainty about the proposed spin-off began to affect HCA's psychiatric hospitals. Physicians and employees were recruited away in what had become a fiercely competitive field. All of the psychiatric hospitals were pressured to fill their beds amid a glut of capacity and increasingly reluctant payers. As the deal lingered, the price dropped. By September 1989, the price tag was down to $1.1 billion, and Frist decided to shop the company around to outside bidders.

Thirty bids came in, including offers by Charter Medical Corp., the second largest psychiatric hospital chain, and two investment banking firms, First Boston Corp. and Morgan Stanley. Charter had just finished a $1.4 billion leveraged buyout by management which eventually jackknifed the Macon, Georgia-based chain into bankruptcy. You can imagine what would have happened had Charter swallowed the $1 billion buy of HCA's psychiatric hospitals.

Meanwhile, Don and his managers put an equity and junk bond financing package together with Kidder Peabody (another New York-based investment banking firm), Bank of Nova Scotia, and General Electric Capital Credit to buy the HCA hospitals. Then in October, the bottom fell out of the junk bond market, sending HCA back to the drawing board.

Next, Don and his team put together a proposal to split up the hospitals: 47 would be put in the new company, while the other 8 to 10 marginal performers would be sold at their real estate value. Still, the price dropped, and the deal lingered, undone.

Finally, in December a savior stepped in. Cigna Corporation, out of Philadelphia, offered to buy HCA's 50 percent stake in Equicor for $777 million in cash. Equicor had been a joint venture between HCA and Equitable Life Assurance Society, out of New York.

With these developments, the pressure was off. Frist could repay the bridge loan with the proceeds and cash from a $545 million recapitalization. He didn't have to sell the psychiatric business after all. Jim Don left the same month to start American Day Treatment

Centers, a chain of day treatment centers for mental health care. The company is based in Baltimore and now markets itself to payers as a cost-efficient alternative to inpatient psychiatric treatment.

Ironically, HCA ended up selling or closing at least half of its psychiatric hospitals, as the mental health business took a nosedive under clouds of scandal in the early 1990s.

Out from under the Equicor arrangement and the bridge loan repayment, HCA forged ahead, striving to focus once again on acute-care hospitals. "We alienated three physicians for every one we pleased," Frist told *Modern Healthcare* (January 2, 1987) in explaining the company's exit from managed care. Nearly everyone started exiting the managed care field, everyone except Humana.

HUMANA CORPORATION STRIVES TO BE THE INDUSTRY LEADER

As much as Thomas Frist Jr. was regarded as an empire builder, Humana's top executives, David Jones and the late Wendell Cherry, were visionaries tempered by business-school priorities. Followers of management guru Peter Drucker, Jones and Cherry studied the ways of IBM and Xerox and molded Humana into a hospital-chain version of those industry titans.

Humana provided the investor-owned industry with lessons in centralization. For example, hospital administrators had to deposit their daily receipts by 3 P.M. Those deposits were then reinvested by Humana's financial leaders by 5 P.M. Humana executives realized the power of the cash flow that the health care industry could generate.

The men were contrarians who took the hospital industry in new directions, never happy with the status quo. "It was addicting working there because you knew you were going to learn so much in the next six months," said a former employee.

Jones and Cherry—two Louisville attorneys—were as close as two business associates could be. Cherry was a sounding board for Jones' ideas and vice versa. Humana was started in 1961 as a nursing home business, Extendicare.

Jones, Cherry, and four other investors each put up $1,000 to get it started. Cherry found the nursing home business depressing, however, and in 1968, the company switched horses to hospitals. After soliciting professional advice, the company's name was changed to Humana.

In January 1968, Jones and Cherry took the Louisville company public at $8 a share. Within 10 months, the price had soared to $50 a share, and the two founders were instant millionaires. Unlike General Care and some of the other hospital chains, Humana didn't enter the joint-venture spree with physicians.

"He [Jones] believed there was a fundamental conflict between doctors and hospitals, and where that existed, it was best not to mix money," said Ira Korman, a former Humana hospital administrator.

HUMANA BECOMES A SHARK

In the early 1970s, Humana grew extensively. Then in 1978, Jones' ambition turned gritty, a characteristic loved by Wall Street. Jones made an unfriendly bid for a much larger company, American Medicorp, a 39-hospital chain. It was the first and last (so far) hostile takeover (a stark contrast to the agreeable deals of the 1990s).

American Medicorp had been nurtured by founders Bernard Korman and Alan Miller. The company's first purchase had been three Northwest hospitals owned by Eugene Brim and two other partners in 1968. Brim had quit American Medicorp in 1971 and had then founded his own Portland, Oregon-based company, Brim & Co., which specialized in contract management for rural hospitals. While at Medicorp, Brim signed what he maintains was the first hospital management contract, with a small hospital in Coos Bay, Oregon.

American Medicorp had pursued an acquisition binge, yet its earnings didn't hold up, and its stock price fell.

Humana's Jones startled Wall Street by offering $19 for American Medicorp stock, which was trading for $1.75. Oddly enough, Trans World Airlines (TWA), a St. Louis-based airline that lusted after the hospital chain's cash flow, upped the ante by offering $24 per share.

Jones never blinked. He offered shareholders $27 to cinch the deal for $305 million. (Medicorp's Miller went on to establish another hospital management company, Universal Health Services, which he still runs out of King of Prussia, Pennsylvania.)

The former American Medicorp hospital administrators met their new bosses for the first time at a meeting in an Indiana hotel across the river from Louisville.

Fresh from the takeover victory, Humana was on a power trip. On the marquee outside the hotel were the words "Medicarp—a Dead Fish." In the hotel's tension-filled meeting room, Jones made a few things clear. "There are only two ways to do things," he told the former Medicorp executives. "The Humana way or get out."

In addition to the facility at Coos Bay, Medicorp had nine other contracts to manage hospitals it didn't own. When an administrator from one of the managed hospitals asked Jones what his fate was to be, Jones answered bluntly, "I never understood how you can make money on managed hospitals, and we don't do what I don't understand." What Jones did understand was how to make money in the hospital business. Between 1970 and 1980, Humana's annual growth rate averaged 32 percent. That exceeded all but eight companies in *Financial World's* performance ranking for companies with revenues of more than $500 million. That same year, Humana was the largest company in the hospital business with 1.4 billion dollars in revenue.

HCA would eventually surpass Humana with the former company's expansion in the mid-1980s. Yet, Jones wasn't interested in sheer size. Employees often heard him say: "Being big is wonderful, but I wouldn't want an elephant to paint my house."

By 1982, an investor who had purchased 100 Humana shares at $8 per share (the initial public offering price) in January 1968 would have had 1,800 shares worth $57,375. Michael LeConey, an analyst with Merrill-Lynch at the time, called Humana the "most aggressive and smartest major company in the United States."

HUMANA AND THE ARTIFICIAL HEART

Despite such accolades from the financial community, for-profit chains lacked the high-quality reputation of some of their not-for-profit peers, such as teaching hospitals. Jones took on that challenge as well when, in 1984, he recruited William DeVries, M.D. from the University of Utah.

DeVries wasn't just any doctor, and Humana didn't have just any plans for him. DeVries was the only surgeon authorized by the Food and Drug Administration (FDA) to perform the artificial heart transplant. He had done the remarkable heart transplantation two years earlier on Barney Clark, but financial and bureaucratic hurdles prevented him from repeating the operation on another patient.

Humana rolled out the red carpet. In essence, company executives told DeVries, "We'll not only pay for you to do a second procedure in this cutting-edge technology, but we'll pay for 100." Humana pledged to donate the hospital care for as many as 100 artificial heart operations at a cost of $100,000 to $250,000 each— an investment of $25 million.

In December 1984, Dr. DeVries and his surgical team at the Humana Hospital-Audubon performed the world's second artificial implant on retired government worker William Schroeder, 52. It was almost a carnival atmosphere in Louisville where the Jarvik-7 heart operation established Humana as the leader in tomorrow's generation of medical wonders. The news was framed by the issue of for-profit medicine, a topic worthy of endless debate around America's dinner tables. For the first time, consumers were talking about whether profit-making corporations should control access to expensive medical procedures such as transplantation, an occurrence that only heightened media interest in the story.

The Louisville Convention Center doubled as a press office, just five minutes away from the hospital. The event—enhanced by handout press photos of Schroeder's discarded natural heart—paid off. Not only did hundreds of newspapers pick up the story, but the surgery grabbed feature articles in the December 10, 1984, editions of *Time, Newsweek,* and *Business Week.* Even *People* magazine came calling (not the kind of publication that usually writes about hospital management types). In the December, 17 edition of *People,* "high-rolling entrepreneurs" Jones and Cherry were profiled, as was Humana's new $50 million headquarters building, which was under construction in downtown Louisville. The article went on to say that critics likened the free artificial heart transplants to free samples of a new product. By giving some transplants away, other critically ill patients would see hope for their conditions in the kind of treatment that only Humana could provide.

Humana generated millions of dollars in free publicity as Americans throughout the country (regardless of whether they had a Humana hospital in their town), now knew the Humana name.

Ironically, the experiment became the first in a series of stumbles for Humana. Schroeder suffered a stroke. Questions about the quality of life for these artificial patients arose, and Humana's motives were questioned. Even so, Dr. DeVries spoke of a higher calling that was consistent with Humana's rarified attitude. In an interview with *The Wall Street Journal* in 1987, Dr. DeVries rationalized the heart operations by quoting dialog from (of all things) *The Wizard of Oz*. DeVries noted that when the Wizard told the Tinman that a heart might make him unhappy, the Tinman replied, "that must be a matter of opinion."

THE HUMANA WAY OF OPERATION

Differences of opinion were not often tolerated at Humana, however, unlike some hospital chains in which individual hospital CEOs could establish their own budget targets, Humana's targets came down from Louisville. Executive directors at the individual hospitals had to meet specific budgets, census day volumes, and profit margins to get bonuses and stock.

Indeed, Humana hospital administrators were known as the best paid administrators in the early 1980s. Humana rewarded them well, tying bonuses and stock awards to profit margins at the individual hospitals. For example, a hospital's executive director could earn up to 50 percent of his or her salary in bonus compensation for meeting the budget, achieving established profit margins, hitting accounts receivable targets, and/or achieving targeted volumes in patient census.

Interestingly, the numbers for bonus calculation were an everescalating target. A case in point; if a hospital administrator's facility made a 20 percent margin one year, Humana would raise the margin 15 percent the next year, and the amount kept going up.

By tying the bonus to profit margin goals rather than dollar profits, the company was structured to grow even during the lean times. For example, an executive director could get a $10,000 bonus for increasing census. However, he or she would receive only $5,000 at the end of the year. The other $5,000 would come in six months, if the hospital's bad debt hadn't gone up. In essence, Humana wanted to ensure that an executive director didn't pack the hospital full of patients who couldn't pay just to get his or her bonus.

To further goad executive directors, the Louisville giant established the Humana Club. Only about one-third of the company's executives earned the coveted club membership, which earned them a two-day trip to Louisville and extra stock. The first year a hospital executive director (ED) made the Humana Club, he or she received 20 percent of the cash value of his or her bonus in stock. However, the Club freshman would only get one-fifth of that stock initially; the rest would be paid over the next four years. The second year the ED made the Humana Club, he or she would receive 25 percent of the value of the bonus in stock. Same formula, though, only one-fifth would be paid the first year. However, the ED would also get another fifth of the first year's stock award.

Each consecutive year an ED made the Humana Club, the percentage would rise by 5 percent to a cap of 55 percent. That tied an executive director to Humana and created incredible pressure to repeat at the Humana Club.

One executive director called this incentive system "velvet handcuffs." There was a distinct penalty for jumping ship. A successful ED who quit might easily walk away from a million dollars or more. Keeping the best, most financially successful executive directors certainly served Humana's bottom line.

The formula worked. In September 1988, HCIA produced a study of the hospitals with the highest operating profit margins in 1987. Of the 40 hospitals with margins of 17.5 percent or higher, 17—almost half—were Humana facilities. Only one of the highly profitable hospitals was a not-for-profit facility. The remaining 22 were investor owned.

Former hospital administrator Korman likened working for Humana to playing for the legendary New York Yankees of the 1960s. As Korman stated, "Nobody liked you, but you didn't care because you knew you were the best."

Humana ran a tightly controlled ship. One example of the stringent control was found in the purchasing area. Most hospitals buy supplies through groups or cooperatives, which receive discounts because they purchase in large volumes. The more a hospital buys, the bigger the discounts. Purchasing groups sign contracts with suppliers, who promise prices based on volume. The groups, in turn, sign contracts with hospitals who commit to buy enough product to obtain the discount.

For example, Hospital A agrees to buy all of its sutures from Vendor A for a certain price. If the hospital buys from Vendor A, B and C, Vendor A is going to be unhappy because it had been promised all of the business.

Compliance to purchasing contracts is the bane of such hospital groups. Regardless of how much the group or cooperative tries to enforce the contracts, individual hospitals often stray. Frequently, a hospital administrator wants to buy a dozen different types of sutures because each of his or her physicians has a different preference.

Humana put a stop to that practice. If Humana signs a contract with one vendor for sutures, that's it. Hospital administrators were allowed to buy only those items for which the company had negotiated discounts.

In 1971, Humana believed it could lower its costs by mandating purchasing contracts. Corporate executives set a goal of 85 percent compliance from individual hospital administrators. Up to that point, compliance had been in the 25 percent range. In other words, only 25 percent of what administrators were buying were supplies on which Humana had negotiated discounts.

To further ensure that this "strongly encouraged policy" wasn't just an exercise in wishful thinking, Humana tied part of administrators' bonuses to compliance. Since Humana centralized its accounts payable function in its Louisville offices, purchasing managers could monitor the extent to which the various hospitals were buying on or off the contracts. If a hospital strayed from the policy, sometimes all it took was a phone call to get them back on the team.

In the first year, the centralized chain achieved an amazing 90 percent compliance—a powerful tool to derive even greater discounts from bandage, aspirin, and intravenous pump manufacturers. After all, a bird in the hand is worth two in the bush. With Humana, vendors had the bird in the hand: a guaranteed volume of sales. Other hospitals only offered two in the bush: more hospital members, but no discipline among the ranks to guarantee sales. Who's likely to get the best prices under that scenario? Intuitively and empirically, the answer was Humana.

This concept of centralized purchasing compliance (as we will see later on in the book) is relevant in the evaluation of contemporary chains. This coalesced clout that a large health care system brings to the negotiating table is one of the distinguishing advantages touted by Columbia executives to achieve a cost advantage over the competition.

HUMANA'S MOVE INTO MANAGED CARE

Jones was smart. Some industry observers even called him brilliant. Importantly, he saw the tide turning. In 1979, charge-based payers had made up 51 percent of Humana's revenues. That percentage was rapidly falling. Consequently, in 1983, Humana launched Humana Care Plus, the forerunner of provider-based managed care plans.

Unfortunately, Care Plus was to become the company's Achilles' heel. To this day, many say that Jones and Cherry had the right idea at the wrong time.

Humana had always had good relationships with its physicians. It had to. Hospitals can't treat a single patient without a physician's signature.

However, its warm regard for physicians became meaningless when Humana started tinkering with two important things: the way they treat patients and they way they are reimbursed.

Traditionally, when a patient was treated, the hospital billed the insurance company, and the physician billed the insurance company. Everybody got paid; everybody was happy.

When Humana became the insurance company, and not just any insurance company, but an HMO, it decided how much the physician would get paid. In many cases, it was offering to pay them less than the physicians had typically received.

This wasn't a foolhardy experiment. The HMO concept had worked for decades for the California prototype, Kaiser Permanente. Yet, here was one big difference. Kaiser's doctors were salaried physicians; Humana's were not.

Like most physicians, Humana's physicians were free agents. There was always another hospital, another insurance company. They didn't have to put up with a company trying to make its mark at their expense.

The launch of Care Plus corresponded with another significant event in health care; the same year, Medicare introduced diagnosis-related groups (DRGs), a prospective payment system in which hospitals were paid a fixed amount, depending on a patient's diagnosis. This new reimbursement arrangement put hospitals at financial risk. The cost-plus days—when Medicare would pay regardless of the costs—were over. This meant length of stay would drop because a significant percentage of hospital business (Medicare and Medicaid) was now reimbursed on a fixed rate. Where would the lost patient days come from?

To survive, perhaps thrive, hospitals needed to be at the top of the food chain. In essence, they needed to be on the receiving end of the premium dollar, doling out payments to the providers, not just receiving per diems or percentage discounts.

Humana was farsighted in seeing the trend. No one was truly "managing" the money spent on health care. Providers sent in the bills, and they got paid, but corporate employers started complaining about how the costs kept rising and rising.

Enter the HMOs. HMOs said they would keep costs in check. Instead of separate charges for the surgeon, the anesthesiologist, the hospital, the pharmacist, and the home health care nurse, an employer would pay the HMO a monthly fee for all services required. The fee would not go up if a patient had a lot of health problems that month. Conversely, it would not go down if the patient made nary a call to his or her physician.

Corporations liked this concept.

In 1983, HMO membership in the United States was 12.5 million. By 1994, membership had grown by more than fourfold, to 50 million individuals. Yet, Jones' vision was marred when the changes foretold for his business didn't come nearly as fast and comprehensively as predicted. It's one thing to set off on a voyage with certain provisions to sustain you until you reach your destination. Still, all the vision in the world doesn't help when the destination keeps stretching beyond your reach.

In Humana's case, timing was off by about five years, but the forecasts at the time were overly optimistic in predicting market acceptance of managed care and other contemporary changes.

A brief look at a few of the forecasts of 1985 demonstrate how absurd they look today. The oft-quoted Wall Street analyst Kenneth Abramowitz of Sanford C. Bernstein & Co., predicted that fee-for-service medicine would be dead by 1990. The respected analyst also predicted that health care costs would drop so drastically that health care would make up only 9.1 percent of the gross national product. Wishful thinking. In fact, health care as a segment of the GNP continued to foment. In 1993, health care hit a new peak—13.9 percent of the gross national product. Although the rate of increase is slowing, it shows few signs of a downward trend.

Abramowitz also predicted major price wars among hospitals by 1987. That, too, did not occur.

Based on such predictions and the market momentum that Humana seemed to possess, coupled with the fact that Jones seemed so certain at the time, most of the big chains followed in his misguided footsteps. It's often said that the hospital industry has a herd mentality. One could offer a textbook case for that thesis with the Humana foray into managed care.

By 1985, HCA and AMI had acquired insurance companies, and NME was shopping for one.

THE INFLUENCE OF INVESTOR-OWNED HOSPITALS ON TAX-EXEMPT HOSPITALS

Not wanting to be left behind, the not-for-profit hospitals joined the parade in getting into the insurance business. In 1983—the same year Humana launched its Care Plus managed care product—Voluntary Hospitals of America (VHA), the nation's largest alliance with 700 not-for-profit hospitals, launched VHA Enterprises (VHAE). Designed to eventually tap the stock market, VHAE dove into several ventures. Fueled by what its executives thought might be an unending source of capital from not-for-profit hospitals, VHAE started individual companies in home health care, mobile imaging, physician search, chemical dependency treatment, medical office buildings, long-term care, and market information.

However, its most expensive venture (and eventually Enterprises' downfall) was Partners Health Plans, a 50-50 joint venture with Aetna Life & Casualty Co., a Hartford, Connecticut-based insurer.

VHAE executives were probably correct when they envisioned managed care as the wave of the future. However, they were not as accurate about other things. For example, VHAE's chief architect, Thomas Reed, vastly underestimated the financial patience required.

"They completely underestimated the amount of time, resources, skills, and personnel it would take to cultivate individual markets," said Sharon Graugnard, president of Preferred Health Management, an Arlington, Virginia-preferred provider organization (PPO) consulting firm.

In 1987, VHA was celebrating its tenth anniversary, yet VHAE was sapping the group's financial strength. Not only was it requiring more and more capital, it was plunging the organization into debt. Acknowledged Mr. Reed at the time, "The expectations for Partners were a lot higher than our ability to deliver."

Mr. Reed was a tall, dark-haired businessman steeped in self-assurance and Wall Street smarts. He seemed to have it all figured out. VHAE could sell its stock at about 18 times earnings. The way he saw it, with just $1 of earnings, VHAE could sell $18 in equity. It then could borrow another $18 against the new equity—giving the company a comfortable 50 percent debt to capitalization ratio. Unfortunately, the nominal $1 in earnings was never realized.

One of the great ironies about VHA is that the strength of the investor-owned chains is what galvanized the group when it was founded in 1977. However, the desire to rip a page from the investor-owned playbook by tapping Wall Street with a public offering threatened the financial security of the alliance itself. What's more, the venture led to the ouster of Mr. Reed and the alliance's first full-time CEO, Don Arnwine. By the time Reed and Arnwine were dismissed, VHAE had lost $87 million on revenues of $305 million.

VHA hired a California hospital system executive, Robert O'Leary, to turn the alliance around. He undid the tangled web of marginal ventures, either selling or closing down each of VHAE's several businesses. With the proceeds from the sale, he paid off VHA's debt of $17.6 million in late 1990 and early 1991. He also paid back the $1.8 million the hospitals had loaned to the alliance in 1983 and 1984 to cover cash flow. The remarkable turnaround of VHA got O'Leary a new job:; president and CEO of American Medical International (AMI).

HUMANA PUSHES ON

VHA got out of the managed care business, as did HCA and AMI. But Humana had made the biggest commitment to the insurance business, and company executives didn't want to admit they were wrong.

One of Humana Care Plus' biggest moves was in the Chicago market, where Humana put the infrastructure in place by buying a financially struggling chain of 29 urgent care centers (now they'd be called primary care clinics) called Doctors Officenters for $17 million.

Humana changed the name to MedFirst Centers. The centers sprouted up in Chicago and other cities where Humana had its Care Plus insurance plan, treating plan enrollees in a less-expensive setting.

In its 1985 annual report, Humana reported that the number of MedFirst Centers had grown from 68 to 148. Humana maintained that by the end of 1986, it would have 350.

Humana was on a roll, and so was Jones. In 1985, *Business Week* reported that Jones was one of the 25 highest-paid executives in the country. He had made $18.1 million in salary and stock options in 1984.

Even so, the business was starting to hemorrhage. In its fiscal year, 1985, the Louisville chain took a $24 million pretax charge on MedFirst and Care Plus development. In Humana's annual report, Jones professed: "Staying the same is easy. Changing, getting better, requires vision, determination and sustained effort."

In its fiscal year, 1986, Humana reported its first year-to-year decline in profits ever, a 75 percent drop to $54 million. It was the company's silver anniversary, but there wasn't much to celebrate.

In October, the once-invincible chain announced it would take a pretax charge of $232 million for its fourth quarter ended September 30, 1986. The amount included after-tax charges of $70 million on Humana Care Plus, $40 million on the sale of 70 MedFirst centers, and $21 million to write down the value of the chain's ill-fated hospital in Mexico City (another grand vision undermined by the plummeting value of the Mexican peso).

In reality, 1986 was the worst year ever experienced by investor-owned hospitals. The big four (led by Humana's disastrous results) reported a $500 million drop in profits.

Ironically, one of the core reasons to start Care Plus was to fill Humana hospitals. But that wasn't happening. In 1986, only 47 percent of Care Plus patients were admitted to a Humana hospital. Humana had planned on capturing 75 percent of the Care Plus business.

In 1987, the 87-hospital chain continued to press on with its managed care strategy, buying a financially ailing Florida HMO, International Medical Centers, for $40 million.

That same year, *Business Week* declared that Jones had "seemed to lose his golden touch." The magazine also highlighted Jones in another way, noting that his pay was the highest, relative to a company's return to shareholders' over the past three years.

While Humana stock waned, Jones had taken in $17.7 million from 1984 through 1986. Most of it came through his exercise of stock options.

Meanwhile, HCA, NME, and AMI were all abandoning their half-hearted ventures into the managed care business. "It looks to me as if there isn't going to be any 'supermed,'" Thomas Frist, Jr. told *The Wall Street Journal* in 1987.

Perhaps the struggles of HCA and Humana were necessary growing pains for a relatively young industry.

"Tommy Frist and David Jones defined the 90s by their actions in the 80s," said Volla. "They were just ahead of their time."

In retrospect, the Humana foray into the managed care/insurance business was significant for several reasons. First, even though the venture proved unprofitable in the early years, it would eventually prove more financially viable than the hospital business.

As mentioned, the concept was sound, but the timing was premature.

Significantly, Humana's commitment to remain in the underwriting arena would eventually polarize the hospital segment and the insurance component—thus leading to the creation of a separate hospital division (known as Galen) and the eventual sale of the hospital segment of the business. Ironically, the move to diversify eventually led to divestiture of Humana's core business: hospitals.

Also relevant is the bitter taste that the Care Plus experience (of the 80s) would leave for the future owners of Galen hospital, namely Columbia. As we will discuss in later chapters, the issue of owning the financing mechanism (i.e. the insurance function) is a controversial and divisive subject for the leaders of today's megafirms.

Humana's Care Plus proved to be not only a bellwether for the for-profits, but a precursor to a highly successful and wildly profitable segment of the industry, the risk-assuming component of health care financing. As fate (or fortune) would have it, where Humana was once chided for its seeming folly, hospitals and health systems now scurry to obtain the mechanism to accept risk and capitated contracts.

Chapter 2

A Rural Return on Investment

When investor-owned chains buy hospitals in rural areas, the dynamics are completely different than those experienced in the city. Out in the country, a hospital may be the largest employer and the only source of medical care for miles around. If it's an investor-owned hospital, it may also be the largest taxpayer in the community.

Not-for-profit hospital executives who berate investor-owned hospitals for not providing enough charity care don't have much to say in small-town America. An investor-owned hospital in that setting has little choice but to take all patients. On the other hand, if the company gets into trouble, the town is going to have trouble. A philosophy of "business knows best" may work in the oil business or the automobile business, but in healthcare, such a corporate attitude can be especially punitive for rural America. If the only hospital in town closes because of mismanagement or financial errors by the corporate chain, the town will suffer the consequences.

For the most part, the big hospital chains that grew in the 1970s and 1980s focused on the city, not the country. For example, in the mid-1980s, HMO guru Paul Ellwood proposed forming a National Rural Health System of America that would band together the purchasing clout of the nation's 2,700 rural hospitals.

Some rural advocates maintained it was a good idea. Some were not as convinced. "Humana and HCA aren't going to be interested in the survival of rural hospitals," said Kevin Fickenscher, president-elect of the National Rural Health Association in a July 5, 1985, issue of *Modern Healthcare*. Obviously this didn't prove to be the case.

Investor-owned hospital chains did become interested in rural systems, but in the late 1980s that experience begot misfortune.

Entrepreneurs tried to duplicate the success of the HCAs and AMIs on a smaller scale. The problem was, rural healthcare didn't pay as well as urban healthcare. The DRG system that proved financially beneficial to urban hospitals was disastrous for many rural facilities. In its initial configuration, Medicare had an urban bias when it came to DRG payments, even though rural hospitals depended more heavily on government reimbursement.

Some rural hospitals depended on Medicare for up to 60 percent of their revenues, yet they received 40 percent less than urban hospitals for the same services.

Why such a discrepancy? Federal actuaries and Medicare reimbursement architects reasoned that rural hospital costs were 40 percent less than their urban counterparts.

They weren't. Health care finance is complex, but it doesn't take a University of Chicago economics scholar to recognize the high percentage of fixed costs involved in a hospital's financial framework. What's more, rural hospital administrators couldn't play the averages in a 40-bed hospital that their colleagues did in a 400-bed hospital. One lingering patient running up $100,000 in bills could send a rural hospital's bottom line south in an instant.

In 1986, Texas led the nation with 18 hospital closures—11 of them were rural facilities. The next year, another nine hospitals closed. Ironically, the closures spurred a search for saviors, which led to new enterprises such as Westworld Community Health Care, Gateway Medical, and National Healthcare.

However, the relief provided by companies such as Lake Forest and California-based Westworld, wasn't necessarily what these hospitals needed. Westworld typically bought the only hospital in a small town, then raised prices two or threefold.

Price gouging allegations took on a life of their own. In South Dakota, the governor warned state employees about high charges at the state's three Westworld hospitals. One example he used was a $15.75 bill for one Tylenol capsule.

Insurers also balked at the stratospheric charges, but Westworld had priorities. Medicare wasn't covering its costs, and the company had 14 percent interest-rate junk bonds to pay off.

Westworld also took Wall Street for an expensive spin around the block, when in 1986, the company's stock fell from a high of $15.38 to 63 cents.

Of the three companies—Westworld, Gateway, and National—only the latter survived the 1980s. National, scarred by shareholder suits and saddled by heavy debt, had pulled all of the tricks in its day, though. At one point, *The Wall Street Journal* described how employees at one National hospital slipped into hospital beds when the company's New York bankers came for a tour so the hospital would seem busier and presumably more profitable.

Apparently the resident administrator reasoned that if there were more patients (even if they were fabricated), the bankers would assume there was more revenue.

THE RISE AND FALL OF A RURAL CHAIN: NATIONAL HEALTHCARE

National's odyssey shows that the hospital industry is not exempt from expert salesmen who can (at least for a while) push all the right financial buttons. The salesman in this case was Stephen Phelps, administrator of Southeast Alabama Medical Center (SAMC), a 400-bed hospital in Dothan, Alabama, before he started National. Dothan was an employee of Hospital Affiliates, which had a management contract to operate SAMC.

When Hospital Affiliates was bought by HCA in 1981, Phelps convinced the hospital's board to give the management contract to him.

That action spawned National Healthcare, which swelled to 28 hospitals by the end of 1985 when it sold $40 million in junk bonds and went public, two financial windfalls shepherded through Wall Street by Drexel Burnham Lambert.

At the time, Phelps was just 35 years old. A year later (1986), *Inc.* magazine ranked National the nation's fifth fastest growing company. *Forbes* featured Phelps in its "Up & Comers" section under the headline "Wal-Mart hospitals."

Forbes didn't coin that moniker, however. In fact, that's how Phelps described his company, "the Wal-Mart of health care." Trouble was, Phelps was no Sam Walton—something that soon became clear to investors and his newly recruited president, Stanton Tuttle.

Tuttle had been a manager at Sears, Roebuck and Company before getting his master's degree in hospital administration at Duke University and racking up more than 15 years of impressive results at Humana, General Care Corporation, and eventually HCA. As president of HCA's psychiatric division, Tuttle was one of HCA's top three executives.

Phelps started calling Tuttle, urging him to come work for National. "I turned him down at least six different times," Tuttle, then president of HCA's psychiatric division, recalled.

Eventually, the HCA executive gave in as Phelps assuaged any fears Tuttle had about the precarious business of small, rural hospitals. "He was as smooth a talker as ever existed...a super, super salesman," Tuttle said.

National's stock was hot on Wall Street. The venerable giants of the hospital industry—Humana, AMI, HCA—were restructuring. National looked like the next good bet for investors.

Unfortunately, the underlying financial status revealed that the company was on very shaky financial footing. National's long-term debt was an incredible 191 percent of equity. Citicorp lent the company $150 million to buy hospitals; instead, National used the loan to pay bills.

When Tuttle joined the company in May 1986, he had no idea the company's financial fortunes were only skin-deep. Between 1984 and 1986, National had purchased 17 rural hospitals and four nursing homes at a total cost of $131 million.

None of these facilities made money. Added to that was the grim reality that National's hospitals were only one-third full, Medicare reimbursement was abysmal, and the company had overpaid HCA for underperforming facilities.

As a condition of his employment, Tuttle was able to recruit his own chief financial officer. He lured Robert Thornton Jr. away from Charter Medical Corporation, the Atlanta-based psychiatric hospital chain. For six months, Thornton and his auditors dove into National's books and reported the results directly to Tuttle. What they found wasn't good. The company had failed to take write-offs for bad debt and Medicare contractual allowances. (Contractual allowances are basically the difference between what hospitals bill Medicare and what they receive in reimbursement.)

Actually, National was losing money. In January 1987, Tuttle took his concerns in writing to the board, urging the company's directors to take the necessary write-offs in contractual allowances and bad debt. Rather than accept Tuttle's recommendations, however, the board listened to Phelps, who convinced the directors to have Thornton report directly to him (Phelps) and the board, rather than Tuttle. Eventually, however, on Sept. 3, 1987, National issued a press release saying that it would report a $19.5 million loss for the fourth quarter, which ended June 1987, citing write-offs for contractual allowances and loan costs as the major reasons for the shortfall.

In another one-paragraph press release the same day, National announced that Tuttle had resigned. The downhill slide accelerated as National faced a $635 million shareholder suit. Phelps resigned from the company, along with three of his vice presidents and two directors on October 1987. At the time of Phelps' resignation, the company's stock was selling for less than 87 cents a share, just a shadow of its $17-per-share price in late 1986.

Under new management, National eventually restructured its debt, selling about $80 million in bonds in 1992 to pay off its bankers.

HEALTHTRUST SWIMS AGAINST THE TIDE

Interestingly, HCA's spin-off, Healthtrust, managed to rise above the woes experienced by National, Gateway, and Westworld. Where these companies faltered, Healthtrust and its top executive, R. Clayton McWhorter, succeeded and subsequently defied the pundits. McWhorter was well acquainted with the rural hospital business, having begun his career as a hospital pharmacist in rural Georgia.

Former President Jimmy Carter—then a state legislator—was one of three members on a committee (in 1965) that hired McWhorter for his first job as a hospital administrator in Americus, Georgia, the same hospital where Carter's daughter Amy was born.

Five years later, Tommy Frist, then executive vice president at HCA, recruited McWhorter to cross the line to investor-owned health care. After some hesitation, McWhorter agreed. Once in the HCA family, the former pharmacist rose quickly through the ranks.

By 1985, McWhorter was president and chief operating officer (COO) of HCA. About this time, HCA stock desperately needed a jolt. Healthtrust was conceived as a way to provide it. HCA executives decided to keep their top 75 hospitals, and spin off the remaining 104 to the employees, in what would be the largest employee stock ownership plan (ESOP) ever.

The ESOP financing for Healthtrust carried huge tax advantages, but that alone wouldn't float the company. It was up to Healthtrust's top managers—Clayton McWhorter, Charles Martin, and Don MacNaughton—to make these underperforming, primarily rural hospitals pay off.

Most of the company's debt carried interest rates of around 10 percent. To ensure that the company didn't sink under its own weight, Frist tossed in three "winners": Eastern Idaho Regional Medical Center—a new hospital (the only one) in Idaho Falls and the largest private facility outside Boise; Bayshore Medical Center in the Houston suburb of Pasadena, Texas; and Plantation General Hospital, a 264-bed facility just outside Fort Lauderdale.

Even these cash cows had some liabilities. For example, Plantation General was located in a highly competitive market that made its profitability status far from a sure thing.

Even though Healthtrust had more acute-care hospitals than HCA (which was now left with 78), HCA's had been far healthier. An analysis by SMG, a Chicago research firm, showed that Healthtrust hospitals only accounted for 39 percent of HCA's patient days.

Healthtrust hospitals were smaller—133 beds on average—compared with 230 beds in the HCA hospitals. The Healthtrust facilities were also emptier: 46 percent full (average occupancy) compared with 59 percent full for HCA's remaining facilities.

The Healthtrust deal was announced in May and immediately the triumvirate (McWhorter, Martin, MacNaughton) started working. MacNaughton was the "gray hair" of the trio, an experienced CEO whom McWhorter could learn from.

"I had always been the operations guy," McWhorter said.

Charlie Martin, the newly formed company's COO, had been in development at HCA and needed to learn the operations of the new Healthtrust hospitals very quickly. Between May and September (of 1985), every Healthtrust hospital administrator came to Nashville to meet with Martin for an hour or two. Martin soon became known for a quick financial mind, attention to details, and a low tolerance for those who didn't work for constant improvement.

"No level of performance was such that it couldn't be improved," Martin said. "With the leverage we had, we didn't have the luxury of being on cruise control."

McWhorter and Martin took on a kind of good cop/bad cop team at Healthtrust. McWhorter was the kinder, gentler CEO who had formerly been the hospital administrators' leader as HCA's COO. Martin was more of a bulldog as the COO of the new company.

Within 18 months of Healthtrust's spin-off from HCA, 60 percent of the hospital CEOs had been replaced. "It's a good incentive," McWhorter acknowledged. Some hospital CEOs didn't even last until Healthtrust was actually formed in September. During the meetings with Martin in Nashville, a few were let go immediately. "A few basically said they weren't interested in working any harder," Martin said.

In the ensuing months, Martin's scrutiny of the hospital CEOs didn't let up. He maintained that "a lot of them didn't seem accustomed to going through month by month, department by department, looking at where the money went." Because most of the Healthtrust hospitals operated in rural communities, Martin could make comparisons, especially for hospitals that were in the same size town or had a similar patient case mix.

Notwithstanding the high turnover, Healthtrust used a carrot as well as a stick for its hospital CEOs. The company increased the incentive compensation, allowing them to earn up to 80 percent of their salary in bonuses.

Meanwhile, McWhorter and others worked on paring away the weakest links. In the next three and a half years, Healthtrust sold 20 hospitals. Interestingly, two of them were in El Paso. They were the first two hospitals purchased by Rick Scott and his fledgling Columbia Hospital Corporation in July 1988. (Making a silk purse out of a sow's ear, Scott turned El Paso into the cornerstone of his now $15-billion corporation.)

In any case, Healthtrust did better without the El Paso facilities. Rural hospitals continued to struggle; 41 of them closed in 1988. Yet, Healthtrust's prospects improved, and in December 1991, the company went public again, raising more than $500 million.

Healthtrust methodically paid down its $2 billion debt burden. By the end of August 1992, the company's debt to equity ratio was 67 percent, down from 95 percent immediately following the spin-off from HCA.

In early 1994, Healthtrust joined the merger sweeps and offered to buy Epic Healthcare Group. Epic had spun off of AMI in September 1988 and never made money. Like Healthtrust, it was financed through an employee stock ownership plan, which gave the firm significant tax breaks. One significant difference between the two companies was that where Healthtrust's Martin kept hospital administrators on a short operational leash, Epic corporate executives gave them free reign.

EPIC HEALTHCARE'S STRUGGLES

Epic and Healthtrust were a study in contrasts. Relations between HCA's Frist and Healthtrust's McWhorter remained friendly from day one of the spin-off. Healthtrust shared information services and group purchasing with its former parent, which owned 10.7 million shares in the spin-off until 1992.

HCA had seemed like family for some of its executives. For example, when Healthtrust shares were languishing in the stock market, McWhorter turned to Frist for advice. Frist recommended Marilyn Herbert, who McWhorter promptly hired as his investor relations director.

Nevertheless, there was a degree of antagonism on the part of Healthtrust executives toward the former parent, which had sent them adrift (in a seemingly ill-equipped craft). Acknowledged McWhorter; "We were just hell-bent that we were going to get up early every morning and beat HCA. If HCA's supply costs per day were a certain amount, we were going to beat it."

Although Healthtrust managers may have manifested some ill-will toward their former parent HCA, it was nothing like the divisiveness that festered between Epic and American Medical International (AMI). When AMI decided to spin off Epic, company officials summoned all the hospital executive directors to Dallas. In a hotel outside the Dallas/Fort Worth International Airport, AMI officials called out the names of 37 executive directors. They were told to go into another room with Kenn George. That's how they found out they were leaving AMI.

George, who headed AMI's southwestern division, was given the top spot to lead the spin-off of Epic. The relationship between Epic and AMI continued to deteriorate. Perhaps AMI's revolving door of executives made any relationship impossible; perhaps Epic wanted to stand on its own. Even after AMI moved its headquarters to Dallas, executives from the two companies didn't visit each other's offices. AMI had a senior executive—Alan Chamison—on Epic's board, but he was mainly keeping tabs on AMI's investment. At one point AMI, which retained a 26 percent stake in Epic, sued company officials over their compensation plan. AMI later dropped the suit, declining to discuss the circumstances surrounding the action.

Under the steerage of Kenn George, a West Texan who walked in cowboy boots and sometimes rode a motorcycle to work, Epic hung on, generating cash, but doing little to wipe off its massive debt load. The company was regarded (by some) as a bunch of cowboys, a sentiment accentuated by the collection of western paintings and sculptures located in the Dallas headquarters. When Healthtrust bought Epic in May 1994, it wasn't surprising that Healthtrust executives gave Epic executives rodeo belt buckles as going away presents. George himself had been a former rodeo rider who gravitated to the oil business in Midland, Texas, before joining AMI. He moved from cutting horses to polo ponies but stayed active in the state's Republican party and was known to harbor political ambitions.

Healthtrust required hospital CEOs to have a management plan and a strategic plan. The CEOs were held accountable for their hospital's financial performance. In contrast, many of the financial functions (such as accounts payable) for Epic hospitals were handled out of the Dallas office. That meant the executive directors (ED) at Epic didn't worry about them as much as their counterparts at Healthtrust.

Healthtrust held seminars on the quality of a hospital's balance sheet. Anyone tampering with their numbers was automatically terminated. Conversely, George's free-wheeling style filtered through the corporate culture of Epic, which stressed employee ownership much more than Healthtrust. Although Epic's hospital

administrators had budgets, insiders said there were few consequences for those who didn't meet them. One executive quipped
that the best incentive was to let a hospital know it was up for sale.
Telling the managers at hospitals in Alice, Texas, and Hope, Arkansas, they were on the sale block produced an "incredible turnaround," he said.

Epic officials also would claim that their hospitals were in worse
shape than Healthtrust's. While Healthtrust was stacked with the
three previously mentioned, large moneymakers, only one of Epic's
hospitals had more than 150 beds, and that one was not exactly a
jewel, as it was slated for sale from the very beginning.

Despite its huge debt burden, Epic had favorable cash flow within
the first six months of the separation from AMI. During that time,
George and his top executives were piling up stock appreciation
rights (known as SARs) that would build in value in spite of the
company's weak financial condition. Unlike stock options that don't
kick in unless the stock reaches a set price, SARs were awarded free
to company executives with no such requirements.

Merger fever hit the hospital chains in 1993, and Epic was regarded by several suitors. However, the company's debt—some of
it financed at sky-high 15 percent interest rates—held many of the
would-be buyers at bay. Even so, the rumor mill got so hot that at
one point in November 1993, George issued a memo to employees:
"Investment bankers are rotating through my office like hamsters
on a treadmill. Every one of them is hot on a deal and sniffing for
a big fee. The perfect deal is just ahead of us! Yeah! Heck, my mother
and father even called with an idea. Gads, people! Go back to
work."

Merger mania filled the air. Healthtrust's McWhorter had been
weighing a bid for governor of Tennessee. When his board insisted
he decide between the gubernatorial race and running Healthtrust,
he chose Healthtrust. Healthtrust was getting offers, but McWhorter
decided to turn the tables. "I needed to take the initiative," he said.

McWhorter and his board offered to buy Epic in January 1994
for approximately one billion dollars. For Epic, it was like manna
from heaven, as well as a godsend for AMI and especially George,
who walked away with $23 million in cash the day of the transac-
tion, largely because of his SARs. AMI cashed in $43 million for its
stake.

The deal bulked up Healthtrust's size by a third, putting it in the big leagues of hospital companies. Once the merger was completed in May of 1994, Healthtrust executives cleaned house at Epic. A condition of the deal was that Epic's top 12 executives would be terminated. Once Healthtrust was in charge, one-third of the hospital CEOs were also replaced. "Bottom line, the company was not very well managed," McWhorter said. "They took their eye off the core business."

Healthtrust's success was proof positive that rural hospitals could be managed successfully by investor-owned chains. Importantly, by the early 1990s, the financial wind was at the backs of rural hospitals. Trying to compensate for past wrongs, Congress put a payment scheme into motion that increased Medicare reimbursement to rural hospitals. That modification—along with a complicated, but financially beneficial geographic reclassification edict—helped rural hospitals become profitable again. In 1992, rural hospitals had a higher profit margin than their urban counterparts.

Interestingly, National Healthcare restructured and changed its name to Hallmark Healthcare. Subsequently (in 1994), the newly-named company sold out to another investor-owned chain that focused on rural and suburban areas, Community Health Systems. By the mid-1990s, Community Health Systems and Health Management Associates had demonstrated success in rural markets, and much of the taint left on small towns by investor-owned firms such as Westworld had faded.

"Most hospital boards today couldn't tell you who Westworld or Gateway was," says Steve Taylor, president of Brim, the Portland-based firm that specializes in managing rural hospitals. That short-term memory, coupled with an attitude change has made rural hospitals fertile ground once again for investor-owned chains in the mid-1990s. "Rural communities used to have the attitude that the hospital was akin to the local high school," Taylor noted. "You wouldn't think about selling the high school," he said, adding, "Now, they view the hospital as a complicated business. Sure, it has social welfare values, but they're (community residents) thinking about it differently."

The main reason this review of investor-owned rural hospital history is highly relevant is that rural hospitals in 1995 may feel insulated from the need to form strategic alliances. The executives at these facilities may not think that Columbia or any other system is interested in their facility due to geographic setting or size. In truth, the merger of Healthtrust with Columbia/HCA should sound a clarion call to small and rural hospitals throughout the country that they are now fair game.

As we have noted, Healthtrust has proven that rural and small hospitals can make a profit. On top of that, with purchaser coalitions being formed in large areas as well as small, the need for extensive geographic diversity is high and increasing. Consequently, the smaller hospitals in the United States (even those located in rural locations) will round out the network for many regional systems. Fundamentally, rural hospitals will need to assess the strategic advantage of alliances and linkages as much as their urban counterparts, if not more so. If the administrators at rural facilities fail to thoroughly evaluate the benefits of increased market leverage available through network involvement, they may find their facility locked out of crucial managed care contracts.

As was pointed out earlier, a fair number of smaller facilities have faced the unfortunate proposition of having to close their doors because they could not compete on cost or breadth of services. Given the increased emphasis on cost containment, that trend will no doubt continue. The hospitals and health systems that will likely weather the storms of reform (market-led reform) will be those that expand their geographic and operational base as well as broaden their financial base and achieve significant economies of scale.

In summary, our prediction is that the stand-alone hospital will not stand alone long. It will either choose to affiliate or (eventually) to disintegrate.

Chapter 3

Reform and the Resurgence of Investor-Owned Systems

Some experts would argue that the for-profit fortunes were made by capitalizing on an attractive arbitrage opportunity. In retrospect, one could argue that the proprietary players entered a market that had operational inefficiencies. They offered a more efficient delivery system on a selective basis, and then sang all the way to the bank.

ARBITRAGE—THE FEDERAL WAY

Arbitrage is, by definition, a financing opportunity that takes advantage of a favorable exchange. It is usually associated with currency rates, but in the case of healthcare, the favorable "exchange" was the financing mechanism of the government, which offered hospitals the unique (and very appealing) prospect of reimbursement on a cost-plus basis. Since the government (via Medicaid and Medicare) typically accounts for between 40 and 60 percent of a hospital's business, this was a no-lose proposition.

Not surprisingly, this mechanism of reimbursement, which Paul Starr noted was, "from the beginning...a recipe for fiscal disaster," was also an irresistible invitation for opportune investment.

The first for-profit hospital chain, American Medical International (AMI), purchased its first hospital in 1960, just a few years prior to the enactment of Medicare legislation.

Correspondingly, the last good year for the investor-owned systems was 1985, just a short while after implementation of diagnostic-related-groups (DRGs), which effectively put an end to the cost-plus formula for government payment. The correlation between the unusual reimbursement rubric instituted by the federal government and the fortunes of the for-profit systems is too direct to ignore. The role of the reimbursement mechanism is also a critical factor in assessing the long-term outlook for the proprietary systems in today's healthcare environment.

Importantly, even the component of healthcare payment not linked to the government—the commercial segment—was not carefully scrutinized by those picking up the tab. Large employers (who account for approximately 80 percent of nongovernment payment) have historically lacked the sophistication and/or interest to closely monitor the payment of healthcare claims.

One of the surprising revelations that surfaced during the debate on healthcare reform was how slowly major corporations had reacted to escalating benefit expenditures and stifling healthcare costs. (Predictably, much of that has changed with the heightened awareness of healthcare as a lead detractor from, or contributor to, the nation's economic engine.)

Significantly, once the market began to adjust to the inherent inefficiency caused by the government's payment system, the phenomenal profits gleaned by the investor-owned chains began to diminish, and the halcyon days of for-profit healthcare rapidly drew to a close. As mentioned, the federal government implemented diagnostic-related-groups (DRGs) in the mid-80s, and as noted, the last banner year for the proprietary systems (up until recently) was 1985. But oh what a ride before the payment path was altered.

Talk to those who started with the chains and experienced their growth from the early days. Many of these fortunate pioneers will readily acknowledge that major mistakes were made, and yet the burgeoning companies continued to make unbelievable profits.

Some companies displayed this "investment invincibility" more than others. Perhaps the consummate case of "conspicuous presumption" was the aforementioned AMI.

Headquartered in the high-rent district adjacent to Rodeo Drive in Beverly Hills, AMI offered (among other corporate niceties) a fifth-floor pastry chef, chauffeured limousines for executives, and stratospheric bonuses for hospital administrators. Despite admitted market misfires with several strategic initiatives, including centralized program administration, a company policy of frequently rotating hospital CEOs, and the now-infamous debacle with AMICare,

AMI continued to prosper financially and operationally. AMICare was the chain's subsequently discontinued venture into managed care.

Indeed, proprietary healthcare was the mother lode in an investment portfolio in the 1970s and early 1980s. In retrospect (based on financial results), one's abilities in operations and administration seemed less important than the concept itself. The key was being a player. As Woody Allen is known to say, "80 percent of success is just showing up." Perhaps in the case of the original for-profit ventures, 80 percent of success was just being in the market with the right model. This was especially true when the market was "subsidized" by a generous underwriter—the federal government— that was willing to provide the capital and payment for services based on development, not demonstrated need.

If we believe that the government had a pivotal role in the genesis of the investor-owned story, we could make the case that activity by the federal government also played a leading role in the resuscitation of the for-profit sector. Perhaps this recent rise in investor prominence was as unplanned as the original impetus.

HEALTHCARE REFORM—PUNDITS AND PITFALLS

When the Clinton administration decided to make healthcare its flagship of domestic policy initiatives, it succeeded in bringing a sensitive issue of concern to the surface. The Pennsylvania senatorial race in November 1991 provided national recognition to the anxiety Americans were feeling regarding access and cost of healthcare, especially cost.

Campaigning on a platform of health reform, Harris Wofford overcame a 40-point deficit in the polls to defeat a former top Bush administration official, Dick Thornburgh. Clinton and his camp attempted to parlay the now-famous Wofford upset into a national rallying cry for healthcare reform, initiated at the federal level. But when Congress rebuffed the Clintons' reformation proposal (with not only a no, but a *health* no!), the stage was set for savvy players to rewrite the script and produce the same (desired) happy ending: reduced healthcare costs.

So, in a sense, even though corporate chieftains such as Columbia's Rick Scott denounce the efforts by the federal government to pursue meaningful reform, it could be argued that the politicos provided both the stage and the audience for the ensuing proprietary performance. In fact, it was shortly after the fruitless efforts of the administration to bring the House and Senate together to pass reform legislation that Rick Scott was hailed as the "Michael Jordan of healthcare reform." You couldn't pay for a better endorsement than that.

Given the tremendous publicity generated about healthcare reform, and this history as a backdrop, one can also better understand why the financial markets have been so excited about recent investor-owned activity. These market watchers remember the mercurial markets of the 1970s and early 1980s and the fabulous fortunes of those insightful investors who banked on proprietary healthcare.

HEALTHCARE—AN INVESTMENT MOTHER LODE IN SEARCH OF A VEIN

Remember also, healthcare is the second largest industry in America, representing over 14 percent of the Gross Domestic Product. Yet, Wall Street has too few vehicles in which to invest in this mammoth industry. Of course, there are the HMO companies, which have had a wild ride on the stock market, and the pharmaceutical and high-tech research or product firms that support the industry. As noted earlier in the book, the significant component (approximately $400 billion) of the trillion-dollar tab belongs to hospital revenues. Add to this over 100 billion that goes to the doctors.

So, over 50 percent of the total is somehow linked to the traditional medical delivery system. This segment alone is larger than most U.S. industries. Yet there remains the dilemma of what vehicle there is for investment.

Enter Columbia. And follow Tenet, OrNda, and the others. Even though the proprietary systems represent only 20 percent of the total number of hospitals, they are an attractive "lightning rod," as investment bankers have termed them, for interested Wall Street investors.

As Figure 3–1 indicates, the for-profit chains had a fabulous ride in the markets in 1993. As it shows, despite relatively "normal"

FIGURE 3–1
Back from the Dead

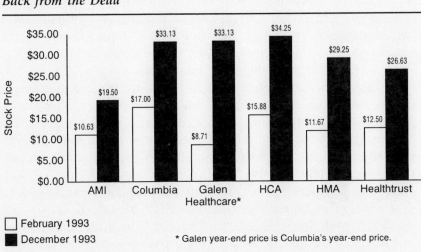

February 1993
December 1993   * Galen year-end price is Columbia's year-end price.

Source: Hospital Networking: Merger Acquisitions and Affiliations, The Advisory
Board Company, 1995 and Donaldson, Lufkin & Jenrette, New York, New York.

earnings performance, the market treated them like a high-tech
Hercules, invincible and insatiable.

SAME SONG, SECOND VERSE?

The $16 billion (revenues for Columbia/HCA) that needs to be
considered by colleagues and competitors is Are the conditions in
the glory days comparable to conditions now? The value of historical (as well as economic) backdrop lies in the comparison of conditions then to what we are seeing in the mid-1990s. Arguably, the
economic winds that propelled the proprietary systems in the 1980s
are somewhat different than those in today's market.

For one thing, the initial foray of the for-profits was characterized
by development of new hospitals with built-in efficiencies, niche
markets, specialized services, and a business orientation. These
dynamics and organizational structures were innovative and intriguing. They marked a change from past practices and policies.
The proprietary program was (as much as anything) a philosophical
shift from the traditional and time-tested view of healthcare delivery in America.

The basic idea was to view healthcare as a business—and run it like one. The oft-quoted axiom of savvy not-for-profits that "You must do well to do good," was basically modified by the investor-owned mavens. In essence, the contemporary credo became, You can do well—in fact very well—by doing good. In this case, the "good" involved the delivery of healthcare.

By taking this business approach to healthcare, investor-owned chains were able to immediately realize economies of distribution and delivery that had not been tested (or exploited as some might say) by the not-for-profit participants who had a slightly different philosophical bent. The very connotation of "not-for-profit" implies that there are other motives for these providers. As the Voluntary Hospitals of America (VHA) recently termed it, a "broader vision." In a widely distributed report, entitled *Realizing the Broader Vision*, the VHA maintained that "Not-for-profit institutions embrace a vision of healthcare that looks beyond profits to broader service to patients and communities." This differentiation of vision (it could be argued), by its very nature places limits on profitability and, understandably, on the amount of effort and attention devoted to the business side of running a hospital.

By focusing on the bottom line, tax-paying executives were able to identify and isolate a core objective that was viewed as incidental by many executives in the industry. This contrast in priorities remains an unbridgeable chasm for many of the veteran administrators in the field. Granted, there are many more hospital executives who have migrated from not-for-profits to for-profits, or vice versa, in the past few years, but there are still many in the masses that divide the two approaches (taxpaying and tax-exempt) with a value orientation, not just a business approach. (This will become a topic of considerable discussion as we explore options for hospitals on an individual basis and as we review case studies of hospital executives who have wrestled with the investor-owned decision).

This divergence of "mission" is a critical notion on which to deliberate, because it lies at the core of the debate—and we think the debate will only polarize the two approaches to healthcare delivery in the next three to five years.

As the proprietary systems grow in size and influence, whatever cordiality existed before will eventually evaporate, and the intensity of the philosophical debate will increase as market competition heats up.

As mentioned earlier, the issue of "arbitrage" is highly relevant. In the late 70s and early 80s, the favorable payment structure coupled with a focus on the bottom line was enough differentiation to contribute to the phenomenal success of the new entrants. This bottom-line emphasis, coupled with the inherent inefficiencies in government-subsidized reimbursement, created an idyllic setting for provider profitability. The healthcare industry allowed ready access and relatively easy expansion for innovators with a different orientation, as well as favorable financing both for services rendered and capital investment and expansion.

Today's market no longer provides easy market entry for new players and new approaches. The unparalleled activity in today's healthcare environment is a result of acquisitions and mergers. The mind-numbing growth of the Columbia system has been an exercise in aggregation, not development. The forces driving this growth are far different than those that propelled the rapid expansion of HCA or AMI in previous decades.

Much of the current frenzy could be attributed to the prominent economic models advanced by the architects of healthcare reform, who maintain that aligned purchasers will require—even demand—provider alliances or networks.

MERGER MANIA AND THE THEORISTS IN THE TETONS

The merger mania of 1993 and 1994 could (along with the political emphasis) arguably be traced to the managed competition model coming out of the Jackson Hole Group (the theorists in the Tetons), who assert that the nation will benefit from consolidation among buyers of healthcare, producing concomitant efficiencies in the costs of delivery. Their market models (such as CalPERS, which negotiates health insurance coverage for California state employees) provide a mechanism for small employers to benefit from the scale of purchasing clout normally reserved for Fortune 500 types.

Their hypotheses also include incentives for providers to offer enough geographic and product diversity to ensure the retention of these large contracts. If there are economies of scale on the purchasing side, so should there be economies on the provider side—both in terms of costs and in terms of distribution.

This consolidation movement on the purchaser side, resulting in parallel alignment on the provider side, is the type of market-led reform that is fundamentally negating the need for politically mandated healthcare reform. As noted in "The Grand Alliance" study by the Governance Committee:

> Report from a dozen markets: Large payer groups now concentrating their business with large-scale providers; over time, classes of smaller players-small insurers, independent hospitals, solo practitioners—in jeopardy of being "locked out."

This market-led reform may in fact produce greater gains on the financial front than those hoped for by the ill-fated political process. The degree of sophistication that is driving consolidation will no doubt bring rationale and reason to the healthcare hydra (i.e., uncontrollable costs) that industry feared and consumers did not understand.

As with the 1970s and 1980s, the driving force behind the proprietary propulsion is fundamentally cost. However, this time, the cost advantage may not be so much a philosophical approach as a systems design.

The concept of large-scale economies (as a means to achieve cost superiority) is perhaps the paramount feature being touted by the market mavens of contemporary medicine. As Rick Scott noted, "We're the largest buyer of medical supplies in the world. We can dramatically reduce their costs."

TWO WAVES—SAME SURF?

The distinction in market dynamics between the two waves of proprietary prominence is highly relevant. There are many who scoff at the recent resurgence of investor-owned systems. Such naysayers speculate that the window of opportunity closed when the healthcare market corrected its inherently inefficient (and singularly diverse payment system). If these pundits are correct, the ensuing consequence would be a sequel to the first roller-coaster ride the for-profits experienced. That saga (mid- to late 80s) of investor indigestion culminated in the stomach-churning depths of despair characterized by the bottoming-out period of the late 80s and early 90s. As mentioned above, most of the growth (to date) by Columbia/HCA could be attributed to acquisition or assimilation. Arguably, the ability to make the behemoth operationally superior and market competitive is yet to be proven. After all, each hospital has a different corporate culture that (Columbia/HCA) must merge. The success or failure of the Columbia endeavor will depend heavily on the economic and operational value of integration.

Importantly, the healthcare market in 1995 is drastically different than that of the prior decade. Purchasers are more savvy. They are demanding greater accountability for increasing prices and decreasing value. There is an unprecedented awareness of healthcare—on Main Street as well as Wall Street. As David Colby, chief financial officer for Columbia/HCA stated last fall, "The system is finally correcting itself. You're getting prudent buyers coming into healthcare. That didn't used to be the case 10 years ago."

With such an awareness comes increased interest as well as skepticism. The purview of physicians is no longer cloaked in intrigue and power, but rather open to public scrutiny and questioning on all fronts. Perhaps this transition in American medicine is the type of environment under which a highly integrated, well-funded delivery system can thrive or even dominate the healthcare market.

Some, like Jeff Goldsmith, have argued that the concept of integration is one that has not been effectively proven in other industries. In an oft-referenced article written in late 1994, in *Healthcare Forum*, Goldsmith notes that "If anything, larger healthcare organizations have actually displayed dis-economies of scale and coordination." He goes on to note that in his experience, systems have "been characterized by more management layers, higher-paid executives, greater dependence on external advisers, slower decision making, and systematic problems relating to those health professionals—such as physicians and nurses—who are in closest contact with the patient and community."

There are certainly enough questions and issues to merit a concerted review of the benefits and potential detriments of aligning with a taxpaying system, which is what we will discuss in later chapters. For now, let us summarize by saying that given the notion that indeed, the past is prologue, the critical question remains is it also analogue?

To the extent you believe the latter premise (that the past is analogous to the present), the direction that hospital boards choose (at least as related to the for-profit systems) will be determined by their prediction of the proprietary market position in the next millennium.

THEN AND NOW—MANY DIFFERENCES, FEW SIMILARITIES

The skeptics in the healthcare theater maintain that the rapid growth of Columbia and the momentum of the for-profits cannot be maintained. In fact, the Mach speed consolidation is, in their opinion, ultimate testimony to the inherent short-term nature of taxpaying prominence. Many pundits argue that the nineties are nothing more than a rerun of the surging seventies for the investor-owned systems.

If such skeptics are correct, the financial and operational doldrums that the original taxpaying chains experienced in the mid- to late 1980s are just around the corner for today's healthcare titans.

Admittedly, there are a few similarities between the market today and the way it was. For one thing, some of the players remain the same: Dr. Thomas Frist, Jr., Clayton McWhorter, Charles Martin ... Interestingly, however, in the case of Frist and McWhorter, even though they are still very much a part of the company they helped develop, their roles have changed. Few doubt that Rick Scott and his lieutenants are very much the lead drivers of the Columbia convoy.

In a way, there is some strategic symbolism to the current configuration of leadership at Columbia/HCA. By keeping these seasoned leaders on board, Rick Scott is making an implied statement that the new order will glean wisdom from the experience of these patriarchs but harness energy and momentum from the young Turks. Not a bad strategy.

Of even more profound significance is the demarcation that separates the old from the new—especially in terms of strategic direction and approach. For the purpose of delineation, allow us to highlight a few of these relevant operational guidelines for the new investment-owned order:

- Cost focused, price driven.
- Decentralized operations.
- Integrated systems strategy.
- Physician position—alignment through incentives.

Cost Focused, Price Driven

Arguably, the taxpaying hospitals have always had a keener sense of cost (on the whole). However, the recent cadre of corporate chieftains are approaching cost from a different angle. When the early investor-owned systems were launched, cost was practically their friend and certainly their facilitator. Hospitals were reimbursed based on cost, so the trick was to utilize costs as an effective facilitator for greater reimbursement.

As has been noted, this was done very effectively by financial experts who came from the insurance industry and who understood the reimbursement mechanism of healthcare.

Interestingly, when the game changed, and Medicare's DRG system of flat rates entered the field, the taxpaying chains weren't much more effective than their tax-exempt counterparts in readjusting to the revised landscape and the revamped ledger. The transition was both sudden and dramatic. The automatic response was to shift the costs to other unsuspecting purchasers of services. At this game, the for-profit executives proved to be all-Pros. Price increases were substituted for innovation or real growth, and for a short time, the shuffling proved effective in maintaining margins and boosting the bottom line—or at least holding it at a respectable level. However, the market soon rebelled at this cost shifting, and all of healthcare came under fire by the public and the purchasers.

Significantly, Scott and his loyal executives have a different starting point and therefore a diverse frame of reference. Their journey along the healthcare highway began in the post-DRG era. For them, cost is neither friend nor facilitator. Rather, the marked emphasis of healthcare strategy in the late 80s and 90s is to monitor and control costs because managed care has made sizable inroads into the delivery system, and these prominent players evoke a "cost is king" attitude.

Symbolically, Scott has publicly championed cost as the most attractive ingredient in his formula for success. From a philosophical standpoint, he has argued that market-led reform is far superior to political reform because it stands a better chance of reducing overall costs in the system. He cites a few of his facilities as proof.

Similarly significant is Scott's position regarding his intention about integrating the insurance component. He has frequently and emphatically stated that his intent is not to enter the financing realm of the system, even if his facilities cannot accept capitation. Scott maintains that he is in the healthcare business, not the insurance or underwriting business. His strategy is to lock in at the low-cost position in every market, so that managed care companies—as well as purchasing coalitions or any buying entity is "forced" to deal with his facilities because of sheer economics. As he states it, "providers will link up with large insurance companies, but Columbia will not pursue the insurance function."

This defined direction is not only indicative of Columbia's emphasis on cost, it also indicates an intense interest in not repeating the mistakes of his predecessors who marched into managed care minefields boldly and returned battered and bruised. Scott and his advisors realize that managed care miscues proved the undoing and/or unraveling of many of the investor-owned systems that attempted to finance the delivery process.

The other investor-owned systems have likely learned from the experience with managed care. For example, AMI was led by executives who either witnessed the debacle of AMICare or, in the case of Robert O'Leary, were responsible for divesting the ill-fated managed care partnership between VHA, the largest not-for-profit hospital alliance, and Aetna Life & Casualty in the 1980s. Understandably, the current executives will not readily venture into the managed care milieu.

AMI and NME, which merged in 1995 to form Tenet Healthcare Corp., have also learned from their predecessors about the relevance of cost. It will no doubt be a long time before the pastry chef is invited to Tenet headquarters.

Decentralized Operations

One of the most important lessons the current leaders appear to have learned is the need to decentralize. Oft repeated is the statement, Healthcare is a local issue, and should be managed at the local level. Of course, nearly everyone accepts that maxim now, but there was a time when the corporate chieftains of hospital chains believed otherwise. As we now know, the light came on for the proprietary pioneers in the mid-80s. Prior to that, the focus of many investor-owned systems was to centralize as many of the operational functions as possible.

As we have noted in comparisons between Columbia and its predecessors, this one important characteristic toward decentralization looms larger than most. Based on our observations, it would appear that the Columbia executives are committed to leaving local leadership in charge. At a panel discussion sponsored by the American Hospital Association in August of 1994, Rick Scott stated that "The success of Columbia/HCA is tied to decentralization—letting local management run the show."

Local administrators of Columbia facilities have far greater decision-making power than their predecessors at HCA, Humana, or AMI. For example, local administrators can hire local architects, something that previously was forbidden at big chains such as HCA and NME. Passing those kinds of responsibilities on to local systems also reduces corporate staff and gives local administrators an incentive to keep a closer tab on costs.

What is perhaps most relevant is the degree of autonomy given individual hospital administrators in setting up local networks. Columbia administrators at the local level are able to tap into regional or national advice, but they have the ability to set up networks with the physicians and with purchaser cooperatives. Although AMI and NME have made great strides in allowing greater autonomy at the local level, they are still not as liberal with authority for local leaders in their system.

Integrated Systems Delivery

Another critical difference between the present proprietary strategy, especially that of Columbia, and the early investor-owned systems, is the attitude toward networks. In the early days of investor-owned systems, hospitals involved in the various corporations were scattered all over the nation, with seemingly little rhyme or reason for location and certainly very little strategic advantage in the regional markets.

Under that structure, the taxpaying chains hoped to gain synergy not from geography, but from corporate strategy, which could (theoretically) be extrapolated from successful hospitals and applied to other aligned hospitals. Given the realization that healthcare is a local issue with local strategies, that centralized approach obviously proved suboptimal.

Columbia has a different tactic and exists in a different environment. In these times, geography is very much a factor. Not only is there hope for synergy, there is a great possibility for symbiosis between complimenting facilities in the same area.

Interestingly, it was this very idea of extensive geographic coverage that purportedly precipitated the merger between HCA and Columbia. Thomas Frist Jr. stated that the realization that all of Florida could be covered by a united system is what converted him conceptually to the idea.

Fundamentally, Columbia has taken the Florida model and exported it to other major metropolitan areas. In doing so, they have broken ranks with the proprietary pioneers, whose strategy seemed to be national in focus. Although Columbia/HCA is very much a national force, it is wielding its prominence market by market or, as Bradford Koles of the Advisory Board terms it, "cobbling together the market at the local level." Figure 3–2 highlights the nature of that initiative in particular regions where Columbia has a strong presence.

As the figure shows, even though Columbia has slightly over 5 percent of the total U.S. market share, it has managed to gain between 20 percent and 40 percent in selected markets.

FIGURE 3-2
National Chains—Local Not National Strategy

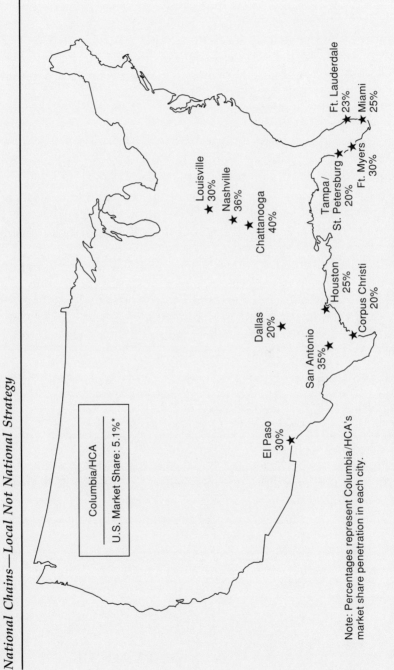

Columbia/HCA

U.S. Market Share: 5.1%*

El Paso
30%

San Antonio
35%

Dallas
20%

Houston
25%

Corpus Christi
20%

Louisville
30%

Nashville
36%

Chattanooga
40%

Tampa/
St. Petersburg
20%

Ft. Myers
30%

Ft. Lauderdale
23%

Miami
25%

Note: Percentages represent Columbia/HCA's
market share penetration in each city.

Source: Hospital Networking: Merger Acquisitions and Affiliations. The Advisory Board Company, 1994

Based on research from that same Advisory Board study, the strategy of pursuing a submarket or MSA network strategy would appear to be the best option. The Advisory Board rated four integration strategies in terms of geographic coverage; its analysis shows that MSA and submarket coverage is far superior to a national or statewide network (See Figure 3–3).

Reverting back to the idea touted by the managed competition gurus that purchasers of healthcare services will band together and form cooperatives, the concept of systems to match the coalitions makes absolute sense. In Florida, the notion was to lock up statewide contracts with employers who have satellites or subsidiaries throughout the state. These multisite companies could contract with Columbia/HCA and not only be guaranteed an established fee, but be assured of consistent treatment protocols and financial coverage for employees of the firms.

The cited difference between large well-known consumer companies and healthcare systems is that (historically) healthcare has been viewed as a terribly personal issue—not like buying hamburgers or garden hoses. In the past, directing employees to designated healthcare facilities or pre-determined physicians was considered un-American, if not unconscionable.

FIGURE 3.3
Geographic Coverage—Choice of Four Strategies

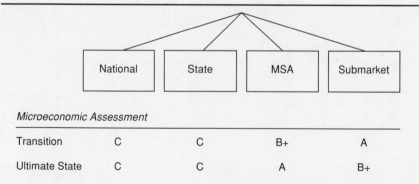

Microeconomic Assessment	National	State	MSA	Submarket
Transition	C	C	B+	A
Ultimate State	C	C	A	B+

Source: Hospital Networking: Merger Aquisitions and Affiliations: The Advisory Board Company, 1995.

But that was before the high costs of healthcare came to the attention of corporate directors and concerned consumers. Importantly, it was also before the notion of coalitions or health insurance purchasing cooperatives (HIPCs), as Paul Ellwood, Alain Enthoven, and the Jackson Hole brain trust termed them.

How many markets or states had large enough businesses to merit a statewide network? (After all, how many university systems, Fortune 500, or state government offices are scattered throughout a given state?) Apparently there were enough statewide purchasing entities in Florida to make the idea attractive to the head of HCA. What's more, the possible networks of small or unaffiliated employers who could join forces either through an employer coalition or through contractual relationships with managed care companies offered the potential for very large numbers of aligned employees.

Consequently, the moves by Columbia/HCA have correlated nicely to the dynamics of the market. The movement toward purchaser consolidation is matched by a similar movement on the supply side—a delivery system capable of geographically and operationally meeting the needs of large segments on the demand side of the equation.

Unlike its predecessors, Columbia believes there are potentially enormous benefits to developing integrated networks at the local level. When Columbia succeeds in upgrading its position from foothold to a strong position in the markets it targets, it becomes a formidable force to reckon with. The effect is that the other players in the field begin to align, and eventually there are two or three systems, where once there were 10 or 12 independent hospitals.

Even if you don't believe in the inherent economies and synergies of aligned hospitals (horizontal integration), the conclusion of the Advisory Board in its recent study on mergers and acquisitions is enough to make you consider the benefits of such a strategy. After conducting extensive research among the leading healthcare systems in the country, the researchers at the Advisory Board concluded that unexpectedly, horizontal integration in the long run will probably not produce the desired cost savings nor strategic advantage. However, the fascinating corollary to that conclusion was the strong recommendation to pursue horizontal integration because it was the best catalyst to achieving vertical integration (alignment with the medical staff). And vertical integration does produce both cost advantages and strategic leverage among nearly all groups of payers.

This latter conclusion is intuitively sound. Physicians are somewhat risk averse. They are interested in aligning with systems or entities that are large by nature and strong in structure. Doctors are more likely to merge their interests and their assets with large-scale networks that offer financial stability and negotiating leverage. Consequently, the consolidation of hospitals into a system will precipitate greater affiliation with previously skeptical doctors. This theory is being proven in markets throughout the country, as doctors choose sides and pick their (large and well capitalized) dance partners.

All of which provides a segue to yet another point of differentiation between the Columbia network and its predecessors: the strategy of aligned financial incentives with participating physicians.

Physician Position—Alignment through Incentives

For a contrast in attitudes toward physicians, you just need to compare some early investor-owned chains with modern-day Columbia/HCA. The fact that Thomas Frist Sr. and Thomas Frist Jr. were both physicians carried over into the HCA corporate attitude toward the medical staff. Physicians were treated with dignity and respect, and they were recognized as the crucial constituency for hospital administrators. Doctors had prominent presence on committees, boards, advisory councils, and policy-making groups at both the corporate and local levels.

Along those lines, HCA was more closely aligned with the traditional administrative methods of dealing with the doctors. Other chains were more businesslike.

Of the contrasting styles, it would appear as though Columbia has adopted the HCA approach, rather than other proprietary predecessors. Scott usually meets with the physicians every time he comes to town. And although it is patently clear he is not intimidated by their stature or their prominence, he is respectful of their profession.

Importantly, Scott and his senior advisors understand the financial architecture of the medical profession and the relevance of aligning the incentives of the doctors with those of the health system—locally as well as nationally.

Consequently, the trademark calling card of Scott and the ubiquitous Columbia representatives is the equity proposition for participating physicians. In the panel discussion at the AHA mentioned earlier, Scott outlined his "operations plan." Significantly, along with decentralization and "high infusion of capital," the salient items of his plan dealt with the physicians:

- Local doctors and management teams buy interest in the facilities.
- Physicians are positioned as co-owners.

Under this innovative (and notably controversial) arrangement involving physician ownership, members of the medical staff can buy up to 15,000 shares in the local system. These shares usually range in price from $10 to $15 so the doctor can buy between $10,000 worth of equity in the Columbia venture or over $200,000 worth of stock, a very intriguing proposition considering some physicians have realized a net gain of 100 percent in less than a year with these arrangements.

This is obviously an offer that is difficult to refuse and one that definitely aligns the critical audience with the newly arrived yet sometimes maligned healthcare neighbor. This strategy could colloquially and appropriately be termed the how to win friends and influence people strategy. And it appears to work marvelously.

To thoroughly appreciate the Columbia/HCA formula, however, it is necessary to review its genesis, which in this case, is a relatively recent occurrence.

Chapter 4

Present Players
Columbia Agitates and Motivates the Industry

As any entrepreneur knows, change breeds opportunity. This is especially intriguing in the healthcare field, where entrepreneurs—both honorable and not so honorable—lurk at every turn.

Among the would-be Waltons of healthcare are doctors, nurses, pharmacists, therapists, billing clerks, and ambulance drivers. If pressed, each can tip an alert investor to some way to turn a buck in this business.

Teeming with cash flow and mismanagement, healthcare is an entrepreneur's paradise. Within a trillion-dollar industry, there's always a better, cheaper way to do something. All you need is the right code so you can bill for it, or so some would argue.

Amid these throngs of entrepreneurs came one more in 1987, Richard Scott, who founded Columbia Hospital Corporation (Columbia). When Scott got into healthcare, hospital companies were out of favor. Doom and gloom filled the air as hospital profits plummeted both in the not-for-profit and investor-owned sectors.

Shareholders who had invested in the big hospital chains were grumbling, and their executives were sweating over restructuring plans.

Presently, Columbia (which, at this writing, is called Columbia/HCA Healthcare Corporation) is the undisputed king of the mountain. Even some consumers are beginning to recognize the company, thanks to a 30-second TV commercial in which Scott himself pledges to cut costs "not a little, but a lot."

Arguably, no one has upset the industry more than Rick Scott. Some pay homage to him as a business genius who's forced the industry to shape up. Others regard him as a profiteer of the sick and vulnerable. Somehow, this 42-year-old former Texan has managed to stir emotions like few others in the industry.

THE COLUMBIA STORY

It's a cold, grey February morning in Louisville, Kentucky, and Columbia Healthcare Corporation is just days away from finalizing its merger with one of the legends of the investor-owned healthcare industry; Hospital Corporation of America (HCA).

Tall and rakish, Columbia's founder, Richard Scott, casually steps from a snow-pocketed parking lot and into the brightly lit lobby of Audubon Regional Medical Center. The building looks like just another suburban hospital in Columbia's growing chain, but it isn't.

This is where Humana made history nearly 10 years before (December 1984), when the world lingered on every heartbeat of William Schroeder, the world's second artificial heart transplant recipient.

At that time, Humana founders David Jones and Wendell Cherry reveled in the media bonfire that spread across the news columns of hundreds of newspapers and magazines. The contrast between the Humana founders and Scott couldn't be more stark. Growing up in North Kansas City, Missouri, Scott used to sit in the back of the classroom so he wouldn't be noticed. He's a proud man, but unpretentious, definitely not Humana-like even though he's taken over all of its hospitals.

On this day in February, Scott seems to feel especially awkward. A video crew is following him around as he roves the hospital, shaking hands with clerks in the admissions department and food handlers in the cafeteria.

He's being taped for an employee video about health reform. Scott smiles often, but never at the camera. He's busy talking to his employees, friendly, not overbearing even though he's obviously the boss here. Who would think this man was recently named one of the "most feared" in the city by *Louisville Magazine*. (Humana founder Jones was voted the "most feared.")

As Scott chats with employees, he hands out a few lapel pins. The one-inch pin consists of the word COLUMBIA in gold, underlined with a red stripe. Scott picked the name himself when starting the company in 1987. It was a name that sounded formidable, and in seven short years, it's grown to fill that description.

Like Scott, the pins are understated, kind of like those diminutive McDonald's signs you see in suburbs where zoning laws won't let the restaurant erect the giant yellow arches. Eventually, the HCA letters will be added to the Columbia pins, making them slightly longer, but little else. Kind of like the company—larger with HCA, but basically unchanged. Even in the combined behemoth that is Columbia/HCA, Scott, his crew, and his strategy remain in control.

When a woman in the cafeteria asks for a pin, Scott discover he's all out. Without hesitation, he reaches up to his own, unfastens it, and offers it to her. She's clearly delighted.

Not everyone is delighted, however, with Columbia's ascent and accompanying clout. The hospital industry still consists of 80 percent tax-exempt hospitals, and the rumblings about Columbia and its mounting clout grow stronger with each passing month. Not-for-profit hospitals don't like his growth, his confidence, or his questions regarding whether their organizations "live up" to their tax exemptions.

Down deep, Scott's detractors believe Columbia will falter. These investor-owned giants always seem to falter: Hospital Corp. of America, Humana, National Medical Enterprises, American Medical International. They stumbled when they got greedy or upset the gods of Wall Street or just got tired of the core business and strayed into unproved territory.

Still, even some of the skeptics wonder, "When will that happen to Columbia? And what if Scott doesn't stumble? What if he just keeps buying and buying and buying?"

Up through 1995, Scott's Columbia had consumed Galen, HCA, and Healthtrust. It is the 800-pound (and $15 billion) gorilla in a $400 billion hospital industry.

"I look at this as a marathon, and we're very early in it," said the 42-year-old lawyer turned health market magnate, whose stake in Columbia is worth nearly $250 million. Now equal in size to health industry giants like Johnson & Johnson and Merck, Columbia is becoming as much a part of consumer's lives as some fast-food restaurant chains.

Columbia's footprints are not nearly as obvious, though. The company is more of a stealth corporation. It owns more than 300 hospitals—Scott has been quoted as saying he wants 500 in 10 years—yet only industry insiders can go from town to town identifying which are Columbia facilities and which are not.

Newly emerged from its acquisition of Healthtrust, Columbia/HCA Healthcare Corporation is the nation's 10th largest employer, a $16 billion company. It's interesting to note how far this industry has come. When Medicare was approved in 1965, all of the hospitals in America together generated revenues of $13 billion. Now, Columbia/HCA, one company with less than 6 percent of the nation's hospitals, generates annual revenues that eclipse that amount.

In just over seven years, Scott has built a company nearly everyone in the industry is talking about. In an October 30, 1994, profile in *The New York Times*, Scott is hailed as "the de facto czar of cost containment" and the "unelected champion of the relentlessly free market." The article itself carries the headline: "Now, It's the Rick Scott Health Plan."

That type of press definitely chafes not-for-profit executives who believe Scott is usurping the credit they deserve for marketplace health reform. In some tax-exempt board rooms, Scott is public enemy number one.

"Up until now, they've just been eating their young," scoffs Mack Haning, a senior director at VHA, the nation's largest alliance of not-for-profit hospitals with 1,000 members. In a VHA publication, the organization refers to Scott as a "zealot." They downplay his influence, saying that not-for-profit hospitals have been doing for years what Scott now grandstands about: consolidation, networking and cost control.

Arguably, much of what they say is true. Rick Scott didn't introduce consolidation to the hospital industry. Nor did he invent the concept of networking among providers. However, he did introduce one element that changed everything in the mid-1990s: speed. Like the runaway bus in the 1994 hit movie *Speed*, Columbia/HCA gave competitors little choice. They had to consolidate or get out of the way. "It appears that I'm changing the industry," Scott says, adding, "All I'm doing is responding to changes in the industry."

As a case in point, look at New Orleans, where three of the city's largest not-for-profit hospitals decided to merge in 1995. Yes, managed care would probably have forced providers to eventually combine their operations, they agreed. However, they looked around and saw Columbia cutting a deal with Tulane University Medical Center, and National Medical Enterprises (NME) negotiating with Louisiana State University's medical center. Peter Betts, president and chief executive officer of one of the three merger partners, East Jefferson General Hospital, commented that "We realized our time frame was a lot shorter because everybody was choosing up sides. We weren't sure there would be partners left to choose from."

SCOTT'S PERSONA EMBODIES COLUMBIA

In the wake of the 1980s era, when hospital managers acted more like colleagues than competitors, Rick Scott's Columbia emerged. In the wake of failed ventures into the insurance business and hospital chains that survived because they just kept raising charges higher and higher, Rick Scott's Columbia flourished. Before Columbia moved to Nashville in 1995, Scott's office in Louisville, Kentucky, overlooked the placid Ohio River, the same river Jones and Cherry likely pondered when building Humana in its halcyon days. The similarities seem to end there.

Humana's corporate headquarters looms over downtown Louisville. When Humana split in two in 1993, the insurance company stayed in the lush corporate offices; and the hospital company, called Galen Healthcare, moved to more modest digs down the street. Humana's stylish $50 million office building, which some locals have dubbed the "Pink Privy," seems an anachronism in the 1990s and certainly contrary to Scott's style.

Humana's headquarters weren't an anomaly among for-profit chains, however. In Beverly Hills, California, AMI's corporate offices at one time were just off the elite Rodeo Drive and featured such executive perks as an in-house pastry chef. "I don't like to spend money," Scott retorted when asked about his plain-vanilla corporate offices. Then, he added, "I don't think I'm going to change."

Kansas physician Raymond Lumb, M.D., recalls visiting Scott's office while considering a deal in November 1994 between his 74-physician group practice—the second largest in the state—and Columbia. Initially, he and his partners had their doubts. "Columbia is so big. There's a lot of fear, a lot of misinformation," Lumb

said. Then, they went to Louisville. "He [Scott] had plastic lami-
nated lamps and a metal file cabinet," said Lumb. Somehow, you
got the feeling that Lumb had been in the offices of plenty of not-
for-profit CEOs whose penny-pinching wasn't as evident.

In an industry that nearly everyone acknowledges wastes millions of dollars every year, Scott's donned the image of a coupon
clipper. In a *Fortune* magazine article in which Columbia was ranked
as the 14th fastest-growing company in 1994, Scott's penny-pinching came out when he revealed that he saves the paper clips from
his mail. Wall Street drools at the potential of what Scott could
wring from a trillion-dollar industry. Savings equal profits; profits
render higher stock prices.

"We're going to be a very volume-oriented company," Scott told
stock analysts in early 1994. Increasing volume means lower costs,
he said, adding, "We want to get ourselves into a position where
everyone wants to do business with us." By demanding discounts
from everyone—cardiac equipment suppliers to head hunters—
Scott believes his hospitals can lower the cost of doing business.
Such a strategy will put Columbia "in a position that no one has
ever been in in this industry," he says flatly. Lindy Richardson,
the company's senior vice president of public affairs, said that
when she has a problem, she tells Scott she wants to talk to some
people to get some ideas. "OK," Scott says, "Talk to some people
in your department." In other words, don't waste money on outside
consultants.

Vendors sometimes complain that Columbia executives are heavy-
handed. The attitude is, in essence, We're Columbia. You can deal
with us on our terms or not deal with us. And, by the way, we want
a discount.

"Part of our success has been that we've been very cost-con-
scious," Scott explains. "We do expect a discount." Scott's call to
cut costs—not a little but a lot, as he says in his multimillion-dollar
TV commercials—couldn't be more timely. Columbia/HCA's rise
coincided with a period of unusually low healthcare inflation. In
1993 and 1994, the medical care component of the Consumer Price
Index rose just 5 percent, the smallest increase in 20 years. Scott
keeps tabs on that index, sending memos to hospital CEOs, remind-
ing them that there's little room to raise charges or costs.

THE FIRST BID FOR HCA

The son of a truck driver, Richard Scott acquired some of his nuts-and-bolts business sense working in a doughnut shop in college. Not much room for wasteful spending when you're charging a buck or two for a dozen glazed.

After graduating from Southern Methodist University law school, Scott joined Dallas' then-biggest law firm, Johnson & Gibbs, in 1977 and began cutting his teeth on healthcare securities, acquisitions, and financial arrangements. After 10 years, he wearied of being on the sidelines, so Scott and two former Republic Health Corporation executives, Richard Ragsdale and Charles Miller, offered $3.9 billion ($47 a share) for Hospital Corporation of America (HCA).

Scott had lined up financing with Citicorp and Drexel Burnham Lambert, which at the time was known as Wall Street's junk bond rainmaker. Even though HCA's board appeared not to take the bid seriously, Scott later maintained: "We were comfortable that all the money was there." Even so, HCA turned the trio down cold. In reflection, "It's funny how these things come around a different way," says Charles Kane, who had been an HCA board member at the time and currently serves on the Columbia board. Ironically, Scott now runs a company that includes HCA. However, at that time, HCA's president and CEO Thomas Frist, Jr., M.D. had no intention of letting HCA fall into other hands.

The trio cordially exited, describing the HCA bid as no more than a "friendly overture." Of that ambitious trio, Scott was the unknown in the industry. Both Ragsdale and Miller were known quantities in the small world of hospital corporations.

Despite his anonymity, Scott had worthy credentials from Ragsdale, Republic's cofounder. Ragsdale later went on to found another hospital chain, Community Health Systems, out of Houston, Texas. Ragsdale knew how Scott, who had been Republic's outside counsel, worked through the night to get Republic's $45 million initial public offering done in 1983. Republic wanted to sell its stock on July 1 before a long Fourth of July weekend. The timing proved fortuitous. Republic stock opened at $23 a share, and never traded higher. The push ensured that Republic raised the most cash.

After the failed HCA bid, life went on for Scott. Miller, however, soon got a call from Fort Worth financial whiz Richard Rainwater. "At first, it didn't hit me who he was," Miller recalls. Then he remembered seeing the former chief adviser to the Bass brothers on the cover of one of the national business magazines. Rainwater, a Stanford MBA, had helped the oil-rich Bass family build its $5 billion empire by dealing in huge chunks of Disney and Texaco stock. He left to start his own investment company in 1986.

"I was referred to you by Tommy Frist," Rainwater told Miller and then explained why he had called. Rainwater wanted to start a hospital company. The idea sounded just intriguing enough to Miller, so he accepted Rainwater's invitation to get together and discuss the idea at a getaway in Nantucket, Massachussets, an old beach motel that Rainwater owned.

"Look, I know Republic had its problems," Rainwater declared. Then he commended Miller on knowing "when to get out," referring to Miller's departure before Republic's ill-fated leveraged buyout (LBO) in late 1986. Rainwater added that he sensed Miller was "smart enough to get off the track before the train wreck." With much to think about, Miller returned to Houston. Finally, he called Rainwater back and turned him down. "I just don't have the appetite to do it again," Miller told him. Rainwater wasn't ready to give up, though. "Can you recommend somebody I can talk to?" he asked. To which Miller responded, "There is a guy I know who is young, smart, sharp, aggressive. His name is Rick Scott."

THE DYNAMIC DUO THAT WOULD CHANGE THE INDUSTRY: SCOTT AND RAINWATER

Rainwater drove to Dallas to visit the potential partner. "The offer was to share an office with him," Scott recalled. The two men would start a hospital company together; no commitment was made about financing. Scott didn't hesitate. He accepted the offer in one day. Somewhat inauspiciously, the Rainwater/Scott partnership began on October 19, 1987, Black Monday—the day the Dow Jones average fell 500 points.

The time wasn't all that great for hospitals either. In 1987, only half of the nation's hospitals made a profit on patient operations. Many were struggling with Medicare's new prospective payment system, which paid them a set price based on a patient's diagnosis. The cost-plus days of charging Medicare were already over.

Medicare margins had been in the 14 percent range in 1984. By 1987, they'd dropped to 5 percent, according to federal figures.

The industry was in a slump, but Rainwater believed the culprit was management, or mismanagement, as the case may be. Both he and Scott saw an opportunity to make a run at the struggling industry. And make a run at it they did. In addition to starting Columbia, Rainwater became an equity investor in American Medical International (AMI), and in 1989 he put up $28 million to help Frist and his managers take HCA private in a $4 billion deal.

Nashville banker and HCA board member Kane remembers having lunch with Rainwater after they had both attended an HCA board meeting and shortly after Rainwater started Columbia with Scott. "He (Rainwater) was talking about the concept and what they were going to do," Kane added. "They felt in the changing healthcare world you needed to be innovative. The concept was good."

To date, Columbia has been Rainwater's most profitable deal. By mid-1994, Columbia was Rainwater's biggest personal holding, according to *Business Week*. Of a nearly $800 million portfolio, his Columbia investment represented $320 million.

Rainwater's wife, Darla Moore, now sits on the Columbia board as Rainwater devotes his time to a new real estate investment trust (REIT) that he started in 1994, Crescent Real Estate Equities. Miller now laughs, saying the biggest mistake he ever made was introducing Scott to Rainwater. Ironically, Miller did get back into the hospital business. His company is Champion Healthcare Corp., a Houston-based firm with nine hospitals. Champion is reviewed in Chapter 5 of this book.

It was Scott, however, who took the initiative in 1987, working from Rainwater's 20th-floor offices on Main Street in Fort Worth. The building was one of two towers sheathed in blue-tinted glass and built by the multibillionaire Bass brothers.

Rainwater's company, Investment Limited Partnership, was full of young Turks, some of whom became millionaires through their ability to buy and sell securities. Regarded as the "Baghdad Bazaar," Rainwater's trading room was full of these men, eyes fixed on computer screens, buying and selling stocks, bonds, even companies. From his office on the 20th floor, Scott did his own buying—of hospitals.

Perhaps no one in the history of hospital management has ever tried so relentlessly to get into the healthcare business as Rick Scott.

In November 1987, Scott wrote 1,000 letters to people he thought might be interested in selling him their hospital. He got no favorable responses. "I tried everything. I called everybody. I flew all over the place," Scott recounted, the frustration evident in his voice. Retelling the experience eight years later, Scott hasn't forgotten how arduous the effort was, especially for a man as impatient as he is.

Married with two school-age children, Scott knew it all hinged on him to get the business underway. Scott went to hospital meetings, dinners, and lunches, hoping to link up with the right people who would open the door to an opportunity...even a crack.

EARLY WINS IN EL PASO

Finally, his tenacity paid off. A group of physicians in El Paso wanted to build a new hospital. Scott talked them out of it. "I told them the more logical thing is we ought to go and try to buy an existing hospital," Scott said.

Logical. Rational. Those are Scott's buzz words, and he uses them at nearly every turn. So, Scott called R. Clayton McWhorter, top executive at Healthtrust. Just prior to Columbia's creation, Healthtrust was formed to take the underperforming castoffs of HCA. Healthtrust was now discarding the hospitals it didn't want. In essence, Scott purchased what some considered the dregs of the industry barrel—two Healthtrust hospitals in El Paso.

To finance the deal, Scott and Rainwater each put up $125,000 and formed a partnership with a group of 110 physicians in El Paso. The partnership bought the two hospitals from Healthtrust, financed with $65 million from Citicorp, in July 1988. El Paso was the maiden voyage and became the prototype for the soon-to-be corporate giant. For Columbia, it was akin to the McDonald's hamburger or the Federal Express overnight letter.

Scott rarely talks about Columbia without mentioning the city where it all began. "What we're going to do is continue to focus like we did in El Paso," Scott often repeats. The El Paso arrangement laid three cornerstones that were the building blocks for Scott's $15 billion company: physician ownership, consolidation, and local market management.

Of the three, physician ownership would be the most controversial. Critics excoriated Scott for trying to buy patient referrals. Yet, he calmly explained that doctors order medical care, doctors de-mand expensive equipment, and doctors significantly influence healthcare costs. By making them financial partners, doctors will think twice before demanding another multimillion-dollar laser or radiology suite. The participating physicians' return (from the partnership) depended on the amount of their investment, not the amount of patient referrals they make, he added.

By and large, doctors are an entrepreneurial breed. They want independence, and they want to be rewarded for their initiative. Arguably, Scott merely tapped into that desire, a desire that some simply dismissed as greed. However, he also tapped into their desire to be part of the decision-making process at hospitals. Some hospital administrators had grown up in the business viewing physicians as adversaries. Rick Scott's approach was, "Let's be on the same team."

All that notwithstanding, a partnership with physicians can be a no-win situation. Often, providers have found that if they refuse to enter into business deals with their doctors, the doctors will simply find another provider that's willing (the any-willing-partner approach). On the other hand, if hospitals do enter a business deal with their physicians, other providers may accuse them of attempt-ing to buy referrals. It's a fine line to walk, yet hospitals that want to survive must find a way to develop a partnership with their medical staff.

Historically, hospitals and physicians have had a somewhat unique relationship. Hospitals are the only business is which people who are not employees—the doctors—can come in and give orders to the employees—nurses, technicians, and so on—and consume their supplies. Oddly enough, administrators and physicians are sometimes at odds with each other in an eternal power struggle. It was kind of an "I need you more than you need me" attitude for both parties.

The dynamics of the present-day market have, however, neces-sitated that hospitals and physicians act in concert (in what is termed "vertical integration") to present a continuum of care as well as an integrated system that can be offered to managed care companies.

In response to the changing needs of the market, and to counter some of the historical divergence between doctors and hospitals, the large chains, including Epic, Healthtrust, and Republic, initiated physician joint ventures, although none with the fervor of Columbia. AMI and NME also tried doctor partnerships but never matched the success of Columbia.

In reality, some physician joint ventures were little more than window dressing. Physicians received a financial stake but not a true say in business. Scott aimed to make his physician arrangements more of a partnership, not just financially but operationally. That's not to underestimate the financial ties. "Physicians are going to be motivated to find alternatives that meet their long-term security needs," noted Denny Shelton, Columbia/HCA's central group president. As physicians' incomes are pressed by managed care payers, they were likely to look for other financially satisfying avenues. Columbia was a boulevard for those.

In Florida's Broward County, Columbia had hoped to raise $16 million in 1994 by selling a 20 percent stake in its network of five hospitals, a home healthcare agency, and a surgery center. To Columbia's surprise, 450 physicians wanted in and were willing to invest $30 million—an amount that would have represented a substantial equity offering on Wall Street. In a sense, Columbia's first partnership in El Paso established the precedent for physician partnerships.

CONSOLIDATION: A CORE CEMENT IN COLUMBIA'S STRATEGY

Another hallmark of Columbia's market strategy occurred in El Paso. After only five months, Columbia bought Landmark Medical Center (a financially weakened hospital that was in danger of losing its Medicare accreditation) for $11 million. The struggling hospital had 355 beds and only 54 patients. Scott promptly closed Landmark and moved the patients over to his other two hospitals. Thus was born another Columbia cornerstone: consolidation.

In El Paso, Scott bought three hospitals and shut one down. Later, in Miami, Columbia merged the operations of Victoria Hospital and Cedars Medical Center, a strategy that might be alien to most hospital management companies. Yet, the consolidation boosted cash flow by $3 million as inpatient and outpatient services were reallocated.

If the government had forced hospitals to merge and close beds, hospital leaders and statesmen alike would have been indignant, screaming about the ominous connotations. Yet in 1994, market-driven consolidation occurred in city after city.

Investor-owned hospitals such as Columbia's weren't the only ones merging. Worried about Columbia, tax-exempt hospitals began looking around for merger partners. Sometimes the parties were motivated by financial considerations—census was dropping and/or HMOs were cutting their payments. However, more often than not, hospital executives and board members were worried about Columbia. Columbia was the straw that stirred the drink. "We're going to liven things up 100 percent of the time when we're in the marketplace," promised Scott's right-hand man, and chief operating officer (COO), David Vandewater.

Another strategy that separates Columbia is its approach to networks or systems in individual markets. In the past, investor-owned chains had been somewhat like corporate vagabonds. They bought one hospital here, one there. Their facilities were spread all over the map. Obviously, for these early systems the priority was not buying hospitals and consolidating them; it was collecting them, building volume and profits. Columbia took a different approach.

Columbia's determination to concentrate on single markets and consolidate hospitals proved a bit risky, though, because a side effect was limiting competition. That ensuing consequence predictably raised the specter of antitrust scrutiny from the federal government—something with which Columbia would become very familiar as the company developed.

This third cornerstone—local market development and management—worked hand in glove with consolidation.

Scott didn't stop with hospitals and physicians in El Paso. He soon opened an 80-bed psychiatric hospital, acquired two outpatient diagnostic centers, and began construction on a three-story cancer center. All of this activity was under the control of a local market manager. "The key is [to] give decision-making power to local management teams. Act like a small company," Scott maintained.

In El Paso, the manager was Russell Schneider, a former Methodist Hospital executive, with seemingly endless energy. Schneider prospered under the authority and autonomy handed him by Scott. Each Columbia market would soon have its own market manager. In Dallas, Scott installed former Humana regional executive Gary

Hill; in Houston, another former Methodist executive, Jay Grinney; in Louisville, former Eralanger Medical Center CEO James Pickle.

Each region had its own president, COO, and chief financial officer (CFO). This represented a new approach, different from the way most investor-owned companies had operated. In traditional for-profit systems, regional vice presidents typically had authority over hospital administrators in their area, yet there was little attempt to work as a team.

Interestingly, Scott structured Columbia/HCA the way HCA had wanted to restructure itself in the late 1980s. In his book, *Management Dimensions*, co-author and then chairman of Healthtrust, Clayton McWhorter, discussed the corporate structure of HCA. The company was divided into four sections: the HCA Psychiatric Corporation, two divisions of owned hospitals, and a division of managed hospitals. HCA had been considering restructuring into one division in which there were four regions, each with its own president; an international division with its own president; and a product specialization division with its own president.

The latter corporate structure is how Columbia/HCA is organized today. McWhorter argued in his book that such a structure would be more responsive to local needs, keeping executives more motivated and enhancing the company's corporate image by keeping operations closer to the markets served. HCA didn't convert to that outlined structure because the resulting upheaval would have been too extensive, McWhorter wrote.

Investor-owned chains too often have operated with layers of mid-level managers, senior managers, and executive managers. In many cases, this bureaucracy left hospital administrators disconnected from corporate management. Additionally, investor-owned hospitals competed for patients and doctors even if they were in the same city and owned by the same company. In retrospect, such a strategy seems incongruous. Yet, it fit the logic of how Wall Street-backed companies operate: living and dying by the quarterly earnings report. The emphasis on quarterly earnings is pushed down to the hospital level and is underscored in the compensation packages for local administrators.

Traditionally, administrators' bonuses were tied to specific hospital performance, not the city, or even regional, system. Helping a sister hospital across town might help the company, but that was irrelevant at bonus time.

Columbia shifted the paradigm. Bonuses hinged on an overall market's financial results, not just a single hospital. Looking at the market in its entirety also provided a big-picture strategy to the entire healthcare system in the region. Under this structure, market managers could appropriately buy surgery centers, home care agencies, or assisted-living centers to fill in the gaps in the healthcare continuum.

Actually, large not-for-profit systems have operated that way for years. Look at Baptist Memorial Hospital in Memphis and its network of hospitals, rehabilitation centers, outpatient centers, a fitness club, and a day care center. For the first time, a tax-paying system, Columbia, was incorporating that strategy into its own plan, and it proved a propitious and profitable one.

Scott instilled his business principles in Columbia market managers and hospital CEOs. Each CEO received a copy of the book *Customers for Life*, by Carl Sewell, a Cadillac dealer in Dallas. Sewell is a meticulous manager concerned about customer perception of quality who built his car lot into a $250 million business. The book includes an entire chapter on rest rooms, for instance. "He says take care of your customers," Scott said of Sewell and his philosophy, adding, "If you do, they're going to be customers for life."

By 1990, Columbia owned 11 hospitals with revenues of $290 million. Profits were a mere $9 million, but Scott was already reporting what would become an industry standard, earnings before depreciation, interest, taxes, and amortization (EBITDA). EBITDA shows a company's cash flow. In essence it's a financial ratio that levels the playing field between not-for-profit hospitals and investor-owned facilities. For example, Columbia reported that the EBITDA generated in El Paso soared upwards from $8.4 million to $40 million in four years.

Meanwhile, in Fort Worth, such financial ratios and other details of proposed deals were sketched out with colorful markers on Scott's floor-to-ceiling, white, vinyl walls. He closely followed stock quotes and stories on his computer and incessantly called physicians and hospital administrators to find hospitals to buy.

In May 1990, Scott had another tool in his financial arsenal, publicly traded stock. Columbia went public through a merger with Smith Laboratories, a San Diego-based medical equipment firm. In keeping with Scott's nature, the merger was actually a frugal way of becoming a publicly traded firm. As an added bonus from the arrangement, he gained $39 million in Smith's cash reserves in the process. Scott frequently criticized the million-dollar fees paid to bankers and lawyers by hospital chains. This merger with Smith Labs was a way to go public and escape a lot of that "wasteful" expense.

Once Columbia was a publicly traded firm, Scott worked hard at meeting the expectations of Wall Street's high-powered stock analysts. Yet, his words often fell on deaf ears. "It was a small company and people ignored it," recalled Jeff Putterman, formerly an analyst at Stephens, a Little Rock, Arkansas-based investment banking firm. "Also, other people in the industry belittled it," Putterman noted.

Correspondingly, some Republic Health Corporation executives privately were accusing Scott of ripping off their company's strategy of physician partnerships. Columbia and Republic were about the same size at that time—medium-sized companies that garnered little attention in the stock market. Stock analysts were paid to research stocks with large shareholder followings, such as National Medical Enterprises and American Medical International. Yet, those who knew Scott saw the momentum building. He wasn't waiting for Wall Street to catch up. "I'm extremely impatient and I try to be results oriented," he explained. In July 1990, Columbia began building its south Texas network, buying HEI, a Houston-based three-hospital chain, for $22 million.

One of Scott's missteps also came in 1990 when he bought Willow Creek Adolescent Center in Arlington, Texas, for $9.4 million in cash and $3 million in assumed debt. Nine administrators later, Columbia sold it to the not-for-profit Adventist system. Remarkably, Willow Creeks's fortunes improved considerably. Administrator Don Sykes said employees threw him a party on his seven-month anniversary with the hospital. No Columbia administrator had lasted seven months prior to his arrival.

FUNDAMENTALLY, A FINANCIAL WHIZ

Not every deal would go Columbia's way. One thing was certain, Scott seemed to excel at raising capital. In March 1992, Columbia sold $100 million in bonds and then in June sold another $135 million to buy Basic American Medical and two AMI hospitals in

Houston for $35 million. By this time, Columbia was named the nation's 12th fastest-growing public company by *Fortune* magazine.

Yet the big transactions, the billion-dollar deals were still around the corner. One day, Stephens' investment banker, Putterman, called Scott and said, "Why don't you ever go to Europe?"

"Nobody's ever invited us to go to Europe," was Scott's answer. Soon the two were jetting across the Atlantic. Stephens hosted a European road show to introduce him to investors over there. "Every time I met with Rick, I came away thinking he was smarter than the time before," Putterman said. Scott was learning from some of the best. One of his smartest moves, he says, was hiring a few men from Methodist Hospital in Houston including Columbia/HCA's chief financial officer(CFO), David Colby.

Methodist was rich and successful throughout the late 1980s and early 1990s. Thanks to sizeable Medicare reimbursement and relatively few charity care write-offs, the 1,500-bed hospital racked up profits of $76 million on revenues of $526 million in 1991. In fact, Methodist was the most profitable hospital in the country that year, according to Healthcare Investment Analyst (HCIA), a Baltimore-based research firm.

The credit for Methodist's stellar performance went to president and CEO Larry Mathis, a brash Texan who ran the hospital like the multimillion-dollar business it was. His management style was so indelibly imprinted on Methodist that some referred to the hospital as "Mathodist."

After agreeing to buy the El Paso hospitals in early 1988, Scott hired two Methodist executives, Russell Schneider and Ruben Perez, to be CEO and CFO, respectively, of Columbia's first two hospitals. Both went out to El Paso in April, yet Schneider stayed in touch with Colby, who was CFO of Methodist. The two men had worked together on an especially difficult financing deal for San Jacinto Methodist Hospital, and respected each other's abilities.

One weekend, Colby went out to help Schneider with Columbia's new El Paso operations. "I didn't make any big secret about it," Colby said. When Mathis found out, he gave Colby an ultimatum. Either stop helping Schneider or stop being CFO of one of the nation's largest and most profitable hospitals. "I'm going to help Russ," Colby answered. He quit Methodist, took one day off, then started the next day for Columbia.

Hiring top executives away from not-for-profit hospitals wasn't the custom among investor-owned chains. They usually recruited from other for-profit companies, or "grew their own," as Humana did, by hiring future managers straight out of graduate school. Still, not-for-profit hospitals are obviously full of strong profit-minded executives. Even though they're called "not-for-profit," over the years these tax-exempt hospitals have been more profitable than their for-profit counterparts. In 1990, for example, for-profits hospitals posted a median total profit margin of 2.5 percent compared with 3.2 percent for not-for-profit facilities, HCIA reported.

The profitability statistic didn't invert until 1992 when investor-owned hospitals reported a 4.5 percent total profit ratio compared to 4.1 percent for not-for-profit organizations. Notably, the gap widened in 1993, when taxpaying hospitals demonstrated a 5.6 percent margin versus 4.2 percent for their tax-exempt counterparts.

Although Columbia has changed drastically in the last five years, the management team has not. Again, that's strikingly different than other investor-owned hospital companies such as AMI and NME, which have had significant turnover at the top.

For example, David Vandewater, has been Columbia's chief operating officer since 1991. Vandewater met Scott through Republic Health Corp., where Vandewater was also COO. Vandewater was very familiar with Columbia's first investment in El Paso, as his first hospital job was running Vista Hills Medical Center (located in El Paso) from 1979 to 1982. Columbia bought Vista Hills in the summer of 1988. Vandewater joined Columbia in July 1990 as senior vice president of operations. At the time, Vandewater acknowledged he was taking a cut in pay from his $300,000-plus salary at Republic. (He would later be handsomely rewarded for his compensation backslide.)

Vandewater remained the number two man behind Scott through all the subsequent mergers. In late 1993, Scott gave Vandewater 109,237 shares of Columbia, worth approximately $3 million. The transaction was an unusual one, a personal transfer of wealth from Scott to Vandewater to thank him for his work in building Columbia.

It's not surprising that Scott's inner circle remained the same while the company grew dramatically in the past few years.

"He knows exactly who his friends were when nobody else was paying attention," said investment banker Putterman. In fact,

Putterman notes that his firm, Stephens, was retained to advise Columbia when it was merging with Galen in 1993. Kind of an odd move since the Little Rock, Arkansas, firm is hardly a Wall Street luminary, such as say, Merrill Lynch or Donaldson Lufkin & Jenrette.

Yet Scott stayed loyal and gave Stephens the business—and a $1.5 million fee. Sounds like a lot, but it's a pittance in Wall Street terms. Galen's adviser, Goldman Sachs in New York, collected $8 million for its advice in the $3.2 billion merger.

Most hospital chain executives didn't blink at the prospect of such fees. Back in 1986, Donaldson Lufkin & Jenrette, another Wall Street investment bank, collected $10 million to advise Scott's former legal client, Republic, in its $800 million leveraged buyout. Despite the high-priced advice, that deal turned decidedly sour as Republic ended up in bankruptcy reorganization. However, the Galen merger sailed along and launched Columbia into the big time. Galen was four times the size of Columbia, bulking up Columbia's once sleek organization.

Up to then, Scott had articulated a simple strategy—expanding the company one market at a time. However, that strategy went out the window when logic dictated another course. Scott had a paper-weight on his desk in Louisville that read: "If you are not the lead dog, the view never changes." What helped Scott move into the lead was a shift among the other "dogs," most notably Humana.

THE GALEN ACQUISITION

Enrollment in Humana's insurance health plan (Humana Care Plus) peaked in 1991 at about 1.7 million. Additionally, Humana's reputation was starting to sag.

Self-promoted as the low-cost providers, Humana was being branded as the high-markup providers. An ABC News report in 1991 slammed the chain for its mark-ups, citing a 60-cent thermometer for which Humana had charged $11.80. Shortly after that occurrence, the Inspector General of the U.S. Department of Health and Human Services initiated an investigation into Humana's Medicare cost reports.

As Humana's star dimmed with the public, the company suffered another crucial blow. In 1991, Wendell Cherry, widely hailed as the company's visionary, died of cancer. The following year, Jones proposed to split the company into an insurance company called Humana and a hospital company called Galen Healthcare (Galen), named for a Greek physician regarded as one of the fathers of medicine.

The move was prompted by the realization that mixing insurance and hospitals was not working. Physicians in some cities, such as San Antonio, rebelled against Humana's managed care plan. In retaliation, they began referring their patients to non-Humana hospitals. Meanwhile, health plans and HMOs that competed with Humana Care Plus didn't want to give any business to Humana hospitals. Humana was burning the candle at both ends.

In the division that ensued, Humana founder David Jones kept the insurance side, which would retain the Humana name. Two long-time Humana executives, Carl Pollard and Jim Bohanon, were named to head the hospital company, Galen.

In March of 1993, Columbia bought a Galen hospital in Beaumont, Texas, and in the midst of talking about other deals, Scott broached the subject of merging with Galen. The deal was simple. Pollard wanted to protect the former Humana employees, so he insisted the merged company be based in his hometown of Louisville. Yet, he basically turned over the reins to the younger and ever-energetic Scott and his team. Bohanon shared COO duties with Vandewater, but only for a few months, at which time Bohanon, a paraplegic with health problems, retired.

The merger with Galen strengthened Columbia's networks in Fort Lauderdale, Houston, and Corpus Christi. Florida was especially important, and soon the company would cover the state like a blanket. (Now, 95 percent of Floridians are within a 20-minute drive of a Columbia/HCA hospital.)

"When Columbia first came to the market, nobody took them seriously," said Miami attorney Sandra Greenblatt. "They were buying hospitals that had never been a competitive threat." Columbia started with another castoff. When Scott bought 300-bed Victoria in December 1988, it was nearly insolvent, losing $400,000 a month. Citicorp anted up again with $17 million, and Scott went into business with 85 local physicians who also purchased equity in the hospital; their individual investments ranged from $20,000 to $30,000. Nine physicians were elected to a Medical Executive Council that met once a week to discuss hospital management. Within a year, the hospital was making money again.

In 1992, Scott bought Basic American Medical, a small Indianapolis-based chain for $185 million in cash and stock. Basic—known as "bammy" for its stock symbol BAMI—derived 80 percent of its profits from a four-hospital network in the Fort Lauderdale area. BAMI's founders had pledged their shares to repay a loan to Marriott and needed to sell. Scott proved to be the white knight they needed.

Through a series of mergers and acquisitions, Columbia grew like kudzu in Florida. "We put down a list of hospitals we wanted to buy," said Vandewater in early 1994, adding, "We've got them." Columbia executives wooed area physicians at a Columbia-sponsored party at St. Petersburg's ThunderDome stadium. Complete with music by a Miami band, the Pink Flamingos, the event cost an estimated $20,000.

THE UBIQUITOUS COLUMBIA

With hospitals and physicians falling in line on a grand scale, Scott was playing a tune that Wall Street loved. The lyrics read "rapid consolidation of a large and fragmented market."

In healthcare, that consolidation was happening in a variety of niches; home healthcare, surgery centers, physician groups, ambulance services. But no other niche carried the clout, the dollars, and the potential for profits as the hospital industry. Suddenly, Columbia seemed to be talking to everyone. The standing joke among hospital administrators was "Have you gotten an acquisition offer from Columbia yet. It's the letter that starts out, Dear occupant."

In city after city, Columbia's acquisition and regional managers pressed forward. They would contact doctors, trustees, and hospital CEOs about selling all or part of their hospitals. They'd send out letters with news clippings about Columbia's latest deals. In Columbia's 1993 annual report, Scott predicted what would happen in 1994, "The shake out has begun, reform is happening and Columbia/HCA Healthcare—not only will we survive—we are positioned to excel."

Indeed, 1994 was to be a banner year for Columbia. It started in February with the $7.6 billion merger/acquisition of HCA, giving Scott and his team control of a $10 billion corporation. "I sought Rick out," Thomas Frist, Jr., noted, in discussing how the merger came about.

However, what Frist never explained was that he was about to radically restructure HCA after he read a copy of the Clinton health plan. Clinton's plan proposed purchasing alliances that would contract with provider networks for care. Columbia's strategy to form networks in local markets made sense to Frist, and he saw it as the future.

Interestingly, Frist's plan to radically revamp HCA was never reported. Frist had planned to convert all of HCA's 100 hospitals to tax-exempt institutions. "I was going to convert six billion dollars in assets and take it off the tax rolls," Frist said later about his grand plan. Goldman Sachs, a Wall Street investment banking firm, was lined up to issue bonds. Frist's plan was to convert all of the hospitals to tax-exempt corporations, but HCA would continue to manage them. Under the new structure, the hospitals could issue tax-exempt bonds, which would be cheaper.

Yet Frist saw a new opportunity with Scott. "Rather than predict the future, you could create the future," he said, regarding his eventual decision to team up with the burgeoning Columbia organization.

Even so, it's curious to think what might have happened had Frist gone ahead with his plan. If HCA had converted all of its hospitals to tax-exempt ones, would other investor-owned chains have followed? As mentioned earlier in the book, the hospital industry is often accused of having a herd mentality. It's highly likely that other systems would have followed HCA's lead. What would that have done to the tax base of the involved communities? Another consideration is whether HCA's move would have led to the demise of the investor-owned hospital sector. No one will know how the market would have reacted to such a dramatic action, but the very fact that he considered such a move demonstrates that Frist thinks big, and he plans ahead for a variety of contingencies. Referring to the plan to convert HCA's hospitals, he commented, "That's the type of contingency plan that's always going on."

This is one contingency plan that remained untested (and largely unknown). Instead, Frist called Richard Rainwater, who was Scott's partner in starting Columbia. Frist had become friends with Rain-water, who had invested in HCA's leveraged buyout in 1988. Frist noted that "Rainwater kept telling me about Rick Scott, and how great he was, and I kept blowing it off." Apparently by 1993, the time was right to heed Rainwater's repeated calls. With the merger, HCA's operations are now in Scott's hands. Frist became chairman, but Scott is "the boss." Two other large mergers followed the HCA alliance. In September, Columbia/HCA bought Medical Care America, the nation's largest outpatient surgery chain, in a $850 million acquisition. Later that year, Columbia initiated the move to merge with Healthtrust.

"It's unlikely I'm going to do anything without Tommy's input," Scott said, when completing the merger with HCA. What the world didn't know was that Frist and Scott were already working together on Clayton McWhorter, chairman, president, and CEO of Healthtrust. In fact, Frist would be pivotal to Scott's dogged persistence in acquiring Healthtrust, which was being heavily wooed by National Medical Enterprises (NME) at the same time.

In January of 1994, one month before the HCA merger was completed, Frist and Scott were already talking to McWhorter about a possible deal. Talks initially had centered around some possible joint ventures or asset swaps, but neither proposition looked good to McWhorter. "Asset swaps are difficult because everyone thinks their assets are worth more," McWhorter said. A joint venture between a Columbia hospital and a Healthtrust facility invariably would put the Healthtrust hospital in a minority position, which wasn't acceptable either.

Talk about a larger deal waned while McWhorter worked to finish Healthtrust's $1 billion purchase of Epic. However, right after that closed in May, Frist and Scott came hounding again. Scott accused McWhorter of procrastinating. "Rick would talk about a price. I would say it's not good enough. Go away," McWhorter recalled.

In early August, McWhorter heard from a new suitor, former investment banker, Jeffrey Barbakow. Barbakow took over NME in 1993 when the company was having deep problems because of fraud allegations surrounding its psychiatric hospitals. Barbakow's job was to turn around the Santa Monica, California-based chain. Barbakow proposed a new tactic: merge Healthtrust with NME and American Medical International (AMI), whose majority owners were looking for a way to cash out. McWhorter agreed to talk, although he was skeptical about whether a final offer would be high enough. Even so, he signed confidentiality agreements with AMI and NME.

By the end of the month, however, Frist and Scott were at the door again, wanting a deal, which provides some insight into how Columbia has completed so many megadeals in the past few years: persistence. Scott and Frist's dogged pursuit of Healthtrust is but one example. Scott and his lieutenants focus on the end goal: getting the deal done. Then, they grit it out. Their determination to do to the deal does not wane.

NME LOSES HEALTHTRUST TO COLUMBIA

In September of 1994, a draft of Barbakow's speech announcing a merger between NME, AMI, and Healthtrust at the annual share- holders' meeting was leaked by a disgruntled employee to *The Wall Street Journal*. It became the biggest whodunit in the hospital indus- try. Who leaked the speech and why? Was the merger going to happen?

While the industry was abuzz with news of a possible triumvirate of NME, AMI, and Healthtrust, Scott and Frist persisted. "Rick's not going to let that happen," said one senior Columbia official when asked about NME's possible deal. The senior official was right.

On September 29, McWhorter held an executive committee meeting at 3 P.M., followed by a board meeting at 5 P.M. He had three options: stay independent, merge with NME and AMI, or merge with Columbia. He considered the numbers and the options. He was going to recommend staying independent.

At 2 P.M., Scott and Frist called. They wanted to up their bid. It was enough. McWhorter walked into the executive committee meeting and recommended the Columbia option. At 5 P.M., the board voted to go with Columbia. Four days later, NME returned with a counterproposal, but McWhorter said it still wasn't good enough. Healthtrust stayed with Columbia.

On October 4, 1994, there was a conference call to announce the Healthtrust deal. On the line were 300 of Columbia's closest follow- ers, Wall Street investment bankers, and analysts. (Quite a change from the days when Columbia couldn't get analysts to write about the company. Now, they were fawning all over the healthcare giant.) All the power brokers were there: Scott, McWhorter, Vandewater, Frist.

Ed Gordon from Morgan Stanley, a New York-based investment banking firm was host. The mood was jovial. Scott introduced everyone. Vandewater was introduced as "the guy who's going to have to pull this whole thing together."

Scott introduced McWhorter as the company's new chairman, adding that Frist—the former chairman—is now vice chairman. Scott joked that "If you're chairman of the board of this company, your longevity is only about six months." McWhorter and Frist were together again.

Putting together billion-dollar deals like Columbia and HCA and Columbia/HCA and Healthtrust takes financial talent—the money has to be right. The chemistry among personalities must be right also. McWhorter and Frist are two guys who can finish each others' sentences. In retrospect, it almost seems ludicrous to think McWhorter would have done a deal with the Californians and New York bankers who run NME.

McWhorter joked that the merger is "an opportunity to rejoin Tommy after being kicked out of the big house and into the condo." He was, of course, referring to Healthtrust's split from HCA.

There's more than a little truth to his jibe. As noted earlier, administrators at Healthtrust hospitals sometimes felt like stepchildren to HCA executives, and relations between the two camps were often tinged with rivalry. With Healthtrust snapped from its grasp, NME, led by Jeffrey Barbakow, was forced to settle for AMI alone. Although Barbakow touted the AMI deal as the best one ever, one Wall Street analyst, Todd Richter, called it an "ego-driven deal. It makes the buyer bigger but not better."

In contrast, analysts loved the prospects of Healthtrust's hospitals joining the Columbia fold. Columbia is a company run by the 40-something crowd. However, McWhorter and Frist add balance from another generation—now regarded as the industry's "gray hairs"— as does Donald MacNaughton, a Healthtrust director and longtime HCA executive who was elected to Columbia's board. MacNaughton, now 77, has been a mentor to McWhorter, 61, and continues in that role.

Following a conference call on the Columbia/Healthtrust merger, MacNaughton talked privately to McWhorter. "You have a problem," he said, flatly. Then he told McWhorter that he had a tendency to talk on too long and that Columbia's president and CEO, Scott, was "going to turn McWhorter off," meaning that at some point Scott might simply stop listening.

McWhorter laughed, and agreed that sometimes he did tend to go on and on in his quest to make a point. He pledged to be quick and concise in his points, especially when talking with Scott, who's naturally impatient. "What I admire most about Don MacNaughton is he tells you what you need to know," McWhorter said.

Columbia now has the men who helped build the investor-owned industry on its board. MacNaughton, Frist, and McWhorter will watch and counsel, but the torch has been passed to Scott, who, at this point, appears to be the race's swiftest runner.

COLUMBIA'S EXPERIENCE WITH NOT-FOR-PROFITS

If Columbia were just buying other for-profit hospitals, it would have been one thing. But Columbia was crossing the tracks, buying not-for-profit hospitals.

"When tax-exempt hospitals look around for a merger partner, I'm the logical person to do business with," Scott says. By selling to Columbia, tax-exempt hospitals could join a network and get 30 percent better prices on medical supplies. That's better than the buying groups of tax-exempt hospitals, Scott argued.

He adds that proceeds from the sale of a tax-exempt facility to Columbia/HCA—usually in the tens of millions of dollars—can fund a host of charitable endeavors in the community.

There are those who question whether Columbia's pricing is indeed 30 percent better, while others wonder if a foundation is better than a tax-exempt hospital. Even so, Scott's arguments are apparently working. In 1994, not a month went by that a not-for-profit hospital wasn't selling out to Columbia or another publicly traded system (a Columbia wanna-be).

Yes, Scott was bringing a mob of emulators with him, aggressive Pac-man capitalists chomping to toss cash towards hospital-selling, tax-exempt boards. It wasn't as easy as Scott made it look, however. Why can't these tax-exempt people make a decision? other investor-owned executives bemoaned.

No chain has purchased more tax-exempt hospitals than Columbia, which ironically, Scott has done while irritating the not-for-profit hospitals as a group. He and his top executives began publicly questioning the tax-exempt hospitals' very reason for being: their mission as a charitable, tax-exempt organization. Scott and his followers believe that hospitals should pay taxes or provide a level of indigent care that makes up for the lack of tax payments. In his mind, it's that simple. Early on, Scott and David Vandewater, Columbia's COO, were clear about how they viewed not-for-profit hospitals. If an individual said "not-for-profit," they immediately corrected him or her. "Tax-exempt," was their corrective reply.

By 1994, the rhetoric was even stronger. "They're not 'not-for-profit,' they're 'non-taxpaying'" was how Columbia's new executives labeled them.

The distinction investor-owned executives make is clear. From their perspective, profits aren't the dividing line between the two classes of hospitals. Taxes are. Some facilities pay them; others don't. That's how the two species differ, they reasoned.

"Non-taxpaying hospitals shouldn't be in business. They're not good corporate citizens," Columbia's Scott said in a 1994 *Washington Post* interview. This quote heard round the healthcare world became a rallying cry for not-for-profit hospital executives. See? I told you this guy was out to get us, they clamored.

Scott contended that his words were taken out of context. In a letter to the *Post*, he wrote: "My comments were focused on the fact that the premise for which non-taxpaying hospitals was established no longer existed, particularly if universal coverage becomes a reality."

Still, nothing really stirred up Scott or his managers more than talking about the labels that historically have described the two distinctions of hospitals. "If we're for-profit, are they for-loss?" Scott asked.

Predictably, Columbia has been accused of playing hardball against tax-exempt hospitals on the issue of taxes. In 1993, the company won a contract away from Lee Memorial Hospital in Fort Myers, Florida, after releasing a study that showed that Lee Memorial was making money on its tax exemption. The study revealed that Lee Memorial was exempted from $10 million in taxes, while only providing $4 million in charity care. That amounted to a $6 million profit on its tax exemption, Columbia charged.

Lee Memorial executives disputed the figures, saying they provided $12 million in charity care and received less than $6 million in tax breaks. Despite the disparity in figures, Columbia won the $7 million contract to provide care to the county's employees.

The Lee case wasn't the end of it, though. The Hospital Alliance of Tennessee volleyed back with a study showing that the state's not-for-profit hospitals provide between 87 and 99 percent of the charity care in their communities. "Who's in control of your healthcare—Wall Street or Main Street?" asked Elliott Moore, the group's president.

"Offers by investor-owned suitors will pale when community leaders understand the benefits of the not-for-profit's commitment to its neighbors and the importance of local control of the services it provides," Moore added.

"Very definitely, there is a stronger division among for-profits and not-for-profits," said John Bozard, vice president for strategic development at Orlando Regional Heathcare System in 1994 after Columbia announced its proposed merger with Healthtrust. Orlando Regional had a joint venture with Healthtrust, but Bozard said that would end with the Columbia merger. "Columbia is a competitor," he maintained, noting the four Columbia hospitals in his region.

The tax status controversy swelled as Columbia pollinated Scott's ideas and funding among the tax-exempt ranks, creating a growing maelstrom of emotions between the tax-exempt and the taxpaying.

By 1995, Catholic leaders also were feeling pressure to speak out. "Not-for-profit healthcare organizations are better suited than their investor-owned counterparts to support the patient-first ethic in medicine," said Joseph Cardinal Bernardin in his address to Chicago's business leaders. "Making the Case for Not-for-Profit Healthcare," in January 1995. "Especially in light of capitation—when providers are at financial risk—the people must ensure that the nation not convert to a predominantly investor-owned delivery system," Bernardin warned.

He warned of "the rougher edges of capitalism's inclination toward excessive individualism," and that the "not-for-profit sector in healthcare may already be eroding as a result of today's extremely turbulent competitive environment in healthcare." Notably, these comments came right after three not-for-profit hospitals in Chicago were sold to Columbia.

Hardly a landslide, but an erosion was under way. Since its acquisition spree began seven years earlier, Columbia has bought hospitals of all religions. It bought a Catholic facility in Fort Worth, Texas; one owned by the Reorganized Church of Jesus Christ of Latter Day Saints in Independence, Missouri; and it merged a Catholic and a Jewish hospital in Miami.

By 1994, other for-profit systems were following the Columbia lead. American Medical International bought St. Francis Hospital in Memphis, Tennessee, for $92 million. Health Management Associates bought Holy Name of Jesus Medical Center in Gadsden, Alabama.

Notably, the number of Catholic hospitals fell from 624 in 1988 to 581 in 1993, according to Catholic Health Association. Scott believes the decline will continue: "It's just logical. Their mission was to take care of charity patients. That mission has passed."

It's interesting how quickly long-time executives at tax-exempt hospitals seem to change their tune, once they're employed by Columbia. In early 1994, James Pickle, president and CEO of Erlanger Medical Center in Chattanooga, Tennessee, was hired to run Columbia's Louisville, Kentucky, hospital network. Despite his tax-exempt roots, Pickle indicted other not-for-profits in Chattanooga, saying that Erlanger—the city's tax-supported public hospital—shouldered nearly all of the city's indigent care. The other not-for-profits in town provided "virtually no charity care," he stated. He further argued that continued tax-exempt status for not-for-profit hospitals was "questionable."

Scott contends that many other public hospital executives agree. He backs his premise up, citing Columbia's acquisition of tax-exempt hospitals in Florida that provided no charity care. Nearly all of the patients are elderly and are covered by Medicare, he explains.

"You're misleading people to say hospitals like Methodist are not-for-profit. It's a joke. They're tax-exempt," said Taylor Boone, who chaired Southwest Texas Methodist Hospital in San Antonio. Methodist agreed to a 50–50 joint venture with Columbia in the early part of 1995 that converted the hospital's tax status to taxpaying and fed about $20 million into a new Methodist foundation. "Methodist has never been 'not for profit,'" he noted, adding that, "it's always made millions of dollars a year in profits."

Boone predicts more and more tax-exempt hospitals will sell to chains. "Some have been part of the problem in healthcare," he adds, citing that the system has become lazy about finding cost-effective ways of delivering care.

Scott isn't a cocky or rude individual. He's unquestionably polite, yet his tendency to say what he thinks, coupled with Columbia's monolithic size, makes his opinions larger than life. This velocity of exposure and expectation can be a detriment. "You don't need to get people bowed up and coming together to depose you," McWhorter recently commented. A case in point: In Houston, one source said the new strategy among tax-exempt hospitals was "ABC—Anybody but Columbia."

Columbia certainly left some disgruntled civic boosters in Louisville, Kentucky. When Scott pulled the company's headquarters out of Louisville 10 months after pledging to stay, locals bad-mouthed him. John Ed Pearce, a columnist for the *Louisville Courier-Journal*, called him "Slick Rick," adding "His heart is on business and is hardened toward civic duties and such. He loves not your city but what he can get from it."

Scott yanked 600 jobs from Louisville, dashing the city's hopes of becoming a healthcare capital, when he moved the company to Nashville. In his defense, Columbia executives claimed the state of Kentucky had not kept its promise to repeal certain taxes.

Additionally, another Louisville columnist, Linda Raymond, reported these insightful comments from University of Louisville associate economics professor, Paul A. Coomes. "Too few business students expect to become entrepreneurs, building a company the way Scott did. After they get their business degrees, they expect someone to hand them a job and a paycheck," Coomes noted. "Scott was a wonderful role model for young people," he added, claiming that he was "a walking, talking, money-making example of what Junior Achievement teaches."

Scott is a capitalist and an entrepreneur whose talents have been both admired and vilified. Scott built a company from nothing, a true entrepreneur. He believes hospitals are businesses. And, he believes they should pay taxes. The question for the future is whether size will be an asset or a liability for Columbia. Largeness may lower overhead costs, but it could raise other less tangible costs.

Columbia has become "Big Corporate Entity" in a business that can be very personal and emotional. When Columbia wanted to close a hospital in Destin, Florida, because it already owned a hospital in nearby Fort Walton Beach, the company was portrayed as an unfeeling monolith. "I think the city is being betrayed," Destin City Councilman Chester Kroeger told *Northwest Florida Daily News.* "We don't want Columbia/HCA in our community anymore."

Under pressure from the state to keep the hospital open by selling it to another buyer, Columbia/HCA agreed to sell it to HMD Healthcare Corporation, out of St. Petersburg, Florida. Coincidentally, HMD's president, Scott L. Hopes, was registered as a lobbyist for Columbia in 1992 when he testified before the Florida Legislature on behalf of a Columbia-commissioned study on physician practice patterns.

Bigness also has disadvantages in getting scores of executives to sing off the same sheet of music. Early in 1995, *Chicago Sun-Times* reporter Della de Lafuente heard from a source that Columbia was interested in buying University of Chicago Hospitals, a powerful 609-bed system. Columbia executives have spoken frequently of pursuing medical school hospitals, and for that reason, the rumor sounded sensible, except for one thing: Columbia already had a relationship with a medical school, University of Illinois, through the chain's largest Chicago facility, Michael Reese Hospital. Still, the source backed up the rumor, saying that Robert Galloway, a Columbia vice president had mentioned a University of Chicago deal in the works during a seminar in Florida. Galloway had spoken at Interhealth, a conference for church-related health systems.

Since most conferences sell cassette tapes of those sessions, de Lafuente called the conference and ordered the tapes of Galloway's session. Sure enough, Galloway mentioned that Columbia either had or was pursuing relationships with five teaching hospitals, and the University of Chicago was one of them. "This would be really big news here," the healthcare business reporter said. "I've got everyone in town looking into this."

The implications were huge. If Columbia bought University of Chicago Hospitals, the chain might not need Michael Reese. Considering Columbia's consolidation philosophy, maybe it would shut the hospital down? The obvious question arose, "How many jobs would be lost?"

Sam Holtzman, who heads the Chicago market for Columbia, finally called back after a few days. "No, no, no," he said. "Galloway doesn't know what we're doing here in Chicago. He just got mixed up because he didn't know the difference between University of Chicago and University of Illinois." That type of confusion could get worse in a company moving at Mach speed and filled with a mix of corporate cultures.

In fact, some pundits question whether Columbia has grown too fast to keep its own operations moving smoothly. "At some point in time, you have to attend to the business," says Robert O'Leary, who formerly headed American Medical International, the Dallas-based hospital chain.

Nonetheless, Columbia's chairman McWhorter was with HCA during its height and says he'll help ensure that Columbia keeps confusion to a minimum by keeping its management structure flat. "You have to be careful about layers," McWhorter said. He further acknowledges that the tough part of a growing company is actually running it. "It's not fun being a captive in your office," McWhorter notes. "It's more fun doing deals and visiting hospitals."

For the myriad healthcare professionals and advisors faced with the daily dilemma of how to deal with the industry giant, *fun* is not likely a word often associated with Columbia.

Consequently, the relevant question regarding Columbia/HCA is, When will the fun run out and, importantly, what will Rick Scott do when it does?

Chapter 5

Present Players
Tenet and Others

Although Columbia/HCA Healthcare Corporation is at the epicenter of this industry's change, other investor-owned companies are stirring up the waters. Some of the more prominent providers are described in the following pages.

TENET HEALTHCARE CORPORATION

Tenet Healthcare Corporation could be Columbia's most formidable adversary in the investor-owned sector. Then again, Tenet could merely become another acquisition target for Columbia.

Formerly known as National Medical Enterprises (NME), Tenet has spent the past few years in a kind of corporate dialysis, purging the impurities from its bloodstream. With the recent acquisition of American Medical International (AMI), the company appears ready to shed its past and go forth anew: an 84-hospital chain with $5 billion in annual revenues. Tenet resulted from the March 1995 merger of NME and AMI. The companies have very different histories although both have their roots in southern California. Tenet remains based in Santa Monica, but its operations center is in Dallas.

Since 1991, AMI had been led by Robert O'Leary, who had no experience with for-profit hospital chains until he was hired by AMI's board in 1991. O'Leary's roots were in the tax-exempt hospital sector, a factor he emphasized repeatedly during his three years at AMI. O'Leary had been president and CEO of Voluntary Hospitals of America, the giant alliance of not-for-profit hospitals based in Irving, Texas.

Basically, O'Leary was brought in to stabilize AMI, both financially and corporately. He followed a revolving door of CEOs. Like

NME, AMI (by 1995) was a small version of a former hospital giant of the mid-1980s. Since the late 1980s, the company had pared down from 118 hospitals to 37, eliminating more than 1,000 corporate and regional positions and piling on $2.2 billion in leveraged buyout debt. At the helm at Tenet is Jeffrey Barbakow who retained only one of AMI's top five executives after the merger. Former COO, John Casey, was kept on—albeit only part-time—to help with not-for-profit hospital acquisitions. Casey brought with him a handful of deals in the works when the merger took place, a welcome addition to NME, which had few or no deals in the works at the time of the merger.

Since coming on board in 1993, chairman and CEO Jeffrey Barbakow has transformed the company's financial and organizational structure while somehow managing to retain the laid-back composure that becomes southern Californians. His background in healthcare is scarce, but he views his role as more of a strategist. "I try to figure out where all this is going," he emphasizes.

Barbakow (a 50-year-old father of two sons) began his financial career as an investment banker at Merrill Lynch in 1969. There he focused on healthcare, media, and entertainment industries, managing debt and equity financings and leveraged buyouts. He was managing director of Merrill Lynch's Los Angeles office when Metro-Goldwyn-Mayer/United Artists Communications (MGM/UAC) tapped him to reposition that company.

After boosting MGM/UAC's cash flow and stock price, he engineered the company's sale in 1991 to Pathe Entertainment Group. Barbakow then became managing director of Donaldson, Lufkin & Jenrette, a Wall Street investment banking firm. Two years later, he took over the top slot at struggling NME. (Interestingly, Tenet's headquarters are just across the street from MGM in Santa Monica.)

His job at NME—now called Tenet—was straightforward. Some industry observers argued that the company had nowhere to go but up; in other words, you can't fall off the floor. However, it could have been worse. Barbakow himself would acknowledge that NME might have been forced into Chapter 11 bankruptcy in late 1993 or early 1994 by its banks if he had not been able to pull the right financial strings.

When it bought AMI, NME decided to change its name to signify its new direction. The name Tenet was chosen from some 1,600 possibilities and carries connotations of high ethical standards and principals. The name is particularly relevant since NME was tarnished in the early 1990s by fraud investigations, lawsuits, and financial losses stemming from its 65 psychiatric hospitals.

Psychiatric care was the downfall of National Medical Enterprises' three founders, all of whom resigned in the wake of allegations that their psychiatric hospitals defrauded patients, insurance companies, and the government. As we quoted NME founder John Bedrosian as saying in Chapter 6, NME was on a growth mission in the 1980s. To an acute-care hospital chain like NME, psychiatric care was an overripe plum just waiting to drop from the branch.

Here's why. Psychiatric hospitals were less expensive to build and cheaper to staff than acute-care facilities. That takes care of the cost side. Now for the revenue side: payment was based on charges rather than fixed-price DRGs. As in the early days of Medicare, providers could charge whatever the market would bear, and insurance companies would pay it. There was little accountability, as the insurers soon found out. Eventually they sued, charging NME with fraudulent billing practices.

Yet, it all sounded very believable at the time. In the late 1980s, some providers were backing up their huge expansion plans with statistics suggesting that one in five Americans has some psychiatric problem and that one in three had an addiction. Even if such statistics were true—which is questionable—it's doubtful that all of those patients needed to be hospitalized. Still, the newly built psychiatric hospitals couldn't turn a profit unless they were filled with patients, and that translated into a somewhat twisted glee on the part of psych managers and employees at finding individuals with mental health problems. Yet, by the early 1990s, everyone—insurers, government officials, consumers, and especially lawyers—was on NME's case.

The day that will go down in infamy for NME employees is August 26, 1993, when hundreds of federal agents surprised NME officials and seized patient records from the headquarters and regional offices. From that point on, much of the company's agenda was determined by the legal ramifications of that wide-ranging federal investigation.

In 1994, NME signed a $379 million settlement with the federal government over alleged fraud in its psychiatric operations. The company has since divested its psychiatric hospitals and rehab hospitals and is focusing on medical/surgical facilities.

Notably, when Barbakow came to NME, the firm had 1,200 corporate employees. Now, Tenet's Santa Monica office has about 100. Another 400 are in Dallas, the operations center for the newly merged operations.

Financially, the company has strong backing, thanks in large part to Barbakow's connections and reputation. To finance the AMI acquisition in March 1995, NME sold $1.2 billion in junk bonds in 1995. Sounds like a lot, and it actually was $200 million more than executives had expected to sell because the demand was so great. NME also received $2.3 billion in bank financing. Interestingly, Barbakow said more than 50 banks were lined up to lend NME as much as $7 billion if he wanted the money.

In the merged entities, Barbakow blended top officials of both firms although most of the senior officials had been with NME. Now called Tenet, the company is switching from the divestiture mode and may become an acquirer of hospitals. Barbakow said Tenet may make a handful of acquisitions each year. The company's debt load won't allow it to become the predator that Columbia is.

Although Tenet is heavily leveraged, Barbakow says the numbers will work out. The company will pay $300 million in annual interest payments and invest $425 million in capital expenditures at the firm's hospitals. The rest should go to the bottom line and subsequently to investors—an arrangement that has bankers and bondholders comfortable with Barbakow. "No excuses," Barbakow says about going forward—the most preferable direction. Surely, everyone at Tenet wants to forget the past.

ORNDA HEALTHCORP

OrNda is the phoenix that emerged from the ashes of Republic Health Corporation (Republic), a Dallas-based company that went through an ill-fated leveraged buyout in 1986. The company recapitalized, restructured, reorganized, and emerged, seemingly revitalized for the 1990s.

OrNda's new start can be marked by the hiring of Charlie Martin, whose roots in this industry trace back to the 1960s and General Care Corporation. Martin rose through the HCA ranks and was one of three key managers chosen to lead the spin-off of Healthtrust in 1987.

Revered for his quick financial mind, yet regarded by some as tempermental, Martin was COO of Healthtrust. Under Martin's tutelage, operating margins at Healthtrust increased from less than 14 percent to 18 percent within two years. They continued to improve to over 20 percent within four years.

Then in September of 1991, Martin left Healthtrust. His four-year stock options had vested, and he was ready to move on. "I was interested in getting where I had a bigger fraction of the action," Martin quipped. He formed his own firm, the Martin Companies, and signed a letter of intent to buy seven hospitals from Safecare. He was in the middle of completing that deal when he got a call from one of Republic's venture capital backers, Paul Levy, who asked if Martin would consider running Republic.

Martin said yes. By January 1992, the 49-year-old industry veteran was back in the saddle, as chairman, president, and CEO of Republic. He brought with him the $125-million deal to buy Safecare and immediately began to analyze Republic's operations and previous strategy. For nearly a year, Martin commuted between Nashville and Dallas. Then in September, he moved the company—which he had renamed OrNda—to Nashville.

Martin wanted to change Republic's name, which carried plenty of negative connotations because of its previous financial woes. Republic's public relations department came up with the name OrNda, an Iroquois term that means "well-being." The word was so foreign to the hospital business that it immediately became the butt of jokes. (In Martin's defense, few of the investor-owned hospital companies can lay claim to having especially imaginative names. Former American Medical International president Royce Diener once related that a university professor told him his company's name was miserable because it consisted of nothing but adjectives.)

Not only did Martin change the company's name and headquarters, he switched strategies. He divested the company's previous diversifications, including surgery centers, clinical labs, and physician joint ventures. Subsequently in 1994, OrNda magnified itself from a small hospital chain to a large one with a three-way transaction. The firm merged with American Healthcare Management (AHM) (a fellow traveler through the bankrutpcy courts) and Summit Health, a small Burbank, California-based hospital chain. The arrangement essentially doubled Martin's company, making OrNda a 46-hospital chain with $1.5 billion in annual revenues. Significantly, OrNda earned respect not previously accorded the rising firm on Wall Street.

Prior to his hiring in 1991, "Republic wasn't on anyone's scale of anything," Martin noted. Now, it's the third largest investor-owned chain, behind Columbia/HCA and Tenet. Jeffrey Villwock, a healthcare analyst for Johnson Rice & Company, a New Orleans-based investment banking firm, believes OrNda will double or triple its size in the next two to three years. "Mr. Martin has come nowhere close to his last acquistion," Villwock said. About three-fourths of its revenues come from hospitals in southern California, Arizona, and southern Florida.

In Arizona, OrNda recently spent $122 million to buy St. Luke's Healthcare System, a not-for-profit system that also owns a Medicaid HMO. Between its California and Arizona operations, OrNda is gaining significant managed care experience, which will work in OrNda's favor. However, on the downside, the company remains among the highest leveraged of the publicly traded hospital companies, with $500 million in floating rate debt, which could be painful if interest rates rise. All of which means Martin and his staff need to keep pressure on OrNda hospital CEOs to perform.

HEALTH MANAGEMENT ASSOCIATES

William Schoen had already engineered one turnaround when he was invited to join the board of Health Management Associates (HMA) in 1983. Prior to that, Schoen had successfully turned around a brewing company, F&M Schafer, and then sold it to Stroh Companies for $120 million. Accordingly, he retreated to Naples in semiretirement.

Kent Dauten, a banker with First Chicago's venture capital division, brought Schoen into HMA and coaxed him to be co-CEO with the company's then-top executive, Joseph Greene. Within two years, Greene was out and Schoen was running the show.

Despite a fickle ride on Wall Street, HMA remains a quiet but consistently successful company. Since going public the second time in 1991, HMA's revenues have nearly doubled to $438 million, and profits have nearly quadrupled to $46 million in fiscal year 1994. Like other investor-owned chains, HMA focuses on purchasing not-for-profit hospitals. However, HMA etches its niche further, concentrating in rural and suburban markets where there is little competition.

The tricky part about operating small-town hospitals, however, is recruiting physicians. Doctors traditionally shun rural areas, but HMA has an edge in recruitment. By having a stable of rural communities to choose from, HMA can give physicians a number of locations from which to choose.

The chain's reputation is nearly spotless. The retired chief executive officer of the nationally famous Mayo Clinic sits on HMA's six-member board—not exactly the kind of industry leader you'd expect governing an investor-owned hospital chain. HMA steered clear of many of the financial gimmicks used by other chains to get ahead. With equity and bank loans, the company has financed a steady growth pattern and accumulated the cash needed to bid for hospitals it really wants.

That doesn't mean HMA executives always get what they want, though. One example of that was Golden Triangle Medical Center in Columbus, Mississippi. This county-owned hospital received 11 offers from for-profit and not-for-profit groups once it decided to sell. Earl Holland, HMA's executive vice president, stood up at the county's board of supervisors meeting and said, "I'll give you $150 million." Recalled Charles Faulkner, the hospital's administrator, "Everybody's britches about fell off." That offer seemed like an enormous sum in a town of around 30,000, yet the board of supervisors said "no." Instead, the board took a lease offer from Baptist Memorial Healthcare System, out of Memphis, Tennessee. That meant the community leaders also said "no" to an additional $800,000 in annual property taxes if HMA had bought the hospital.

All of which goes to prove that for some people (especially in smaller communities) money isn't always the deciding factor. We'll discuss this point in greater detail in the latter part of the book, but the Columbus anecdote provides a good case study to corroborate that premise.

COMMUNITY HEALTH SYSTEMS

In 1982, the newly elected mayor of Troy, Alabama, Jimmy Lunsford, proposed that the city sell its hospital, 97-bed Edge Regional Medical Center. What was the reaction? "I was the biggest scoundrel in town," Lunsford proclaimed. Yet the new mayor thought it made sound economic sense. He reasoned that the city could sell the hospital at a profit and stop subsidizing the facility to the tune of about $500,000 a year. Even so, nobody wanted to give up their town hospital.

Twelve years later, Community Health Systems (Community), a Houston, Texas-based hospital chain came to Lunsford with an offer to buy the hospital. Lunsford sat on it, mulling it over for two months without telling anyone. When he finally presented the proposal, there was "virtually 100 percent support" from the town of 15,000 residents.

So what was different? Managed care was on the horizon. Edge Regional was getting emptier and emptier, despite the town's best efforts to improve the physical plant and recruit physicians. Recruiting doctors was the hardest part. "You can be in the nicest facility in the world, but if you don't have doctors..." Lunsford said, not finishing a sentence that had an obvious conclusion. In 1992, the hospital averaged 38 patients a day. One year later, the census had slipped to 35. By 1994, the hospital averaged only 30 patients a day.

Baptist Medical Center, located about 50 miles to the north, also had offered to acquire the hospital—for free. "They offered nothing," Lunsford noted. On the other hand, Community offered $14 million.

Troy is the perfect example of a Community Health Systems hospital. Although the town's population is only 15,000, the hospital's service area is larger—some 40,000. Importantly, Edge Regional is a sole community provider, which means no local competition. Community focuses on markets with population ranging from 20,000 to 60,000. Of the chain's 40 hospitals, 26 are sole community providers.

Generally, Community acquires hospitals that have been getting about 30 percent of the healthcare dollars in town. It's not unusual for a rural hospital to get that much; the other 70 percent goes to hospitals in other larger towns or cities. "Our goal is to get 50 percent," says Deborah Moffett, Community's CFO. One way to do that is to recruit more physicians. Rural physicians have always been notoriously hard to recruit, but Community's size helps. As with HMA, Community can centralize recruiting costs and efforts.

Although Community has been around since 1985, the company hit the big leagues in 1994, when it bought Hallmark Healthcare Corporation. Formerly called National Healthcare, the company was a rural hospital chain discussed in Chapter 2. Community's purchase of Hallmark doubled the number of hospitals it operated to 40, spread throughout 17 states. Community finished 1994 with $466 million in revenues.

BRIM & ASSOCIATES

One of the oldest hospital management companies, Brim & Associates (Brim) concentrates on managing rural hospitals. Founder A. E. "Gene" Brim is one of the industry's pioneers, who began developing hospitals in 1963 with two partners. In December 1968, the partnership sold its three hospitals to American Medicorp, a firm that had been started just seven months earlier. It was the first acquisition for American Medicorp, which was scooped up in a hostile takeover by Humana in 1978.

Brim initially stayed on to run the hospitals for Medicorp but left in 1971 because the company wasn't putting the promised capital into the facilities. He then started A.E. Brim & Associates, a consulting service that soon expanded into a management contracting company. "It was a product whose time had come," Brim declared.

By 1973, the company was managing five rural hospitals in the Northwest. In 1980, the fledgling firm, seeking a well-capitalized partner, was sold to a tax-exempt organization, Fairview Community Hospitals of Minneapolis. However, the Fairview partnership fell apart because Brim had increasing capital requirements, and Brim executives became impatient at the not-for-profit's slow decision-making process. In 1984, Hillhaven, the nursing home subsidiary of National Medical Enterprises, bought Brim, and both companies looked to expand into medium-sized and small communities. By 1986, Brim was also managing NME's 15 hospitals that were under management contracts.

In yet another restructuring at NME, the company sold Brim in 1987. In February 1988, Brim and its officers repurchased the company, which remains privately held. Like Quorum, Brim got into purchasing hospitals but lacks the capital to buy as many as Quorum. Still a privately held company, Brim manages 64 hospitals and 14 retirement centers. In mid-1995, Brim agreed to merge with Paracelsus Healthcare Corp.

QUORUM HEALTH GROUP

In HCA's post-LBO divestiture days, the Nashville-based company spun off Quorum. Quorum was HCA's management subsidiary, meaning that it had contracts to manage not-for-profit hospitals that were owned by others. Frequently, the others were local governments. However, since its spin-off from HCA and subsequent public offering, Quorum Health Group (Quorum) has expanded into hospital ownership as well. By 1995, Quorum owned 11 hospitals and had agreements to buy two others, both large systems.

Quorum is led by a core of former HCA executives who spent their early years driving down country roads where their customers—small, rural hospitals—were located. Although Quorum bought its first hospital in 1990, the company established itself as a true wheeler-dealer in 1993 when it bought 10 acute-care hospitals from Charter Medical Corporation for $340 million. Almost acting as a broker of hospitals, Quorum's president and CEO James Dalton kept just four of the 10. The rest were sold, closed, or traded in a series of transactions during 1994.

In May 1994, Quorum raised $100 million in its initial public offering. Quorum continues to manage 260 hospitals—four times more than its closest competitor, Brim. Like Brim, virtually all of Quorum's managed hospitals are owned by tax-exempt organizations or governments. The average management fee was $179,000 in 1994. With numbers like that, it's easy to see why many hospital companies don't fool with management contracts. It's much more profitable to own hospitals than merely manage them.

Managing hospitals in rural America is an interesting business, though, which throws the company into the thick of small-town politics time and again. The management and strategic direction of Baylor University Medical Center in Dallas or Barnes Jewish Christian in St. Louis rarely makes the newspapers. Not so for a small county-owned hospital that's managed by a large out-of-town corporation.

Hospitals in small towns are often the largest employer, and if they're public hospitals the board meetings are open to the community. Small-town newspapers, where eager journalism neophytes often cut their teeth, are frequently ready to pounce on a hospital controversy—and Quorum has found itself in the midst of more than one.

For example, in tiny Livingston, Texas, a ballot initiative on whether to increase tax support to a Quorum-managed hospital, Polk County Memorial Hospital, nearly split the community apart. In the weeks leading up to the May 1993 election, the semiweekly *Polk County Enterprise* was chock-full of stories, full-page advertisements, and letters to the editor from both sides. The opposition was organized and vocal. At one point, the group attacked two hospital executives for spending a whopping $946 to attend a two-day Quorum management meeting in Las Vegas.

W.O. "Zero" Lewis, a local resident who opposed the new tax, took out a full-page newspaper ad attacking the tax increase. "Polk Countians have been polarized by this Quorum plan and Quorum's political agenda," he charged. The vote failed although Quorum has won tax elections in other small towns.

Notably, these types of management contracts aren't nearly as profitable as owning hospitals. Quorum's revenues have grown six-fold to $641 million between fiscal 1991 and 1994, thanks to the newly acquired hospitals.

Quorum is looking for the same type of hospitals as Community Health Systems and Health Management Associates. Dalton and his staff target hospitals with between 100 and 400 beds in towns with 50,000 to 400,000 residents. Of the nation's 5,300 hospitals, about 1,200 meet that profile, Quorum informed shareholders in its 1994 annual report.

Although other chains have bought more not-for-profit hospitals, Quorum hasn't been any slouch. It bought the first Baptist hospital sold to an investor-owned chain—Baptist Memorial Hosital in Gadsden, Alabama, for $70 million in 1993. The firm's most recent acquisition is a Lutheran Hospital in Fort Wayne, Indiana, whose proposed sale is protypical for perhaps hundreds of hospitals.

Fort Wayne is a three-hospital town. All three had been not-for-profit hospitals. The largest, Parkview Memorial, has about a 40 percent market share; the remaining 60 percent is evenly split between Lutheran and St. Joseph Medical Center. At one point, Lutheran talked to St. Joseph about a merger, but negotiations broke down over religious issues (such as sterilization), a common occurrence in Catholic hospital mergers.

This presented a dilemma. Obviously, Lutheran couldn't merge with Parkview. The resulting 70 percent market share would draw a strong challenge from the Federal Trade Commission on antitrust grounds. If Lutheran wanted to join a system, and thereby gain the benefits of group purchasing, access to capital, and managed care expertise, it had to go outside Fort Wayne. It found Quorum.

The change in ownership will be something new for Fort Wayne— a tax-paying hospital.

UNIVERSAL HEALTH SERVICES, KING OF PRUSSIA, PENNSYLVANIA

Alan Miller founded Universal Health Services (Universal) in 1978 after Humana, with a hostile bid, bought his previous hospital chain, American Medicorp. Universal stands apart from the other hospital companies in several ways. Universal is kind of a one-man show with Miller at the helm. A former Army captain, he controls it financially and, although it's a publicly held company, it's the least public of the investor-owned chains.

The company has four classes of stock. Miller owns 92 percent of the Class A stock and 91 percent of the Class C stock. The Class B stock, which is the only class that is publicly traded, is more widely dispersed, although Miller owns 1.2 million shares—a 9 percent stake. However, the other classes of stock can be converted at any time into class B stock, giving Miller considerably more clout. What's more, he holds 82 percent of the voting power.

Clearly, this unique structure would seem to indicate that Miller never wants to go through another hostile takeover like the one he experienced with American Medicorp.

Miller's top lieutenant, Sidney Miller (no relation), controls another 6.5 percent of the voting power. So, while the public stock owns three-fourths of the equity in the hospital chain, it has less than 10 percent of the voting power.

Many other hospital chain CEOs are the embodiment of their companies: Scott is Columbia, Schoen is Health Management Associates, and so forth. Yet, none has the control that Miller exerts over Universal.

Another unique aspect to Universal's underlying capitalization is its real estate investment trust (REIT). Wanting to reduce its debt, Universal launched Universal Health Realty Income Trust, using money raised from a public offering to buy 11 Universal hospitals. Universal used the money to pay down debt but has to make monthly lease payments to the REIT. Despite assurances that it would diversify its portfolio of properties, the REIT continues to depend on Universal's hospitals for 90 percent of its revenues.

Although Miller bristles at comparisons, that was a recipe for disaster for another hospital chain and its REIT. Healthcare International in Austin also sold most of its hospitals to its own REIT, HeathVest. Like Universal, Healthcare International provided advisory services to its REIT. Other healthcare REITs aren't "self-advised," meaning that independent managers determine what properties to buy and at what price. However, the ultimate downfall of HealthVest and Healthcare International was that the REIT paid too much for its hospitals. Miller says that's not the case for Universal's REIT.

Universal owns 26 hospitals, 13 of which are psychiatric. However, two hospitals have accounted for nearly all of the profits in recent years: McAllen (Texas) Medical Center, which made a $42-million profit in 1992, and Valley Hospital Medical Center in Las Vegas, which made a $26 million profit in 1992. Universal as a company had a profit of just $20 million in 1992.

Ironically, McAllen is located in one of the poorest regions of Texas, along the U.S.–Mexico border. Even so, the area is booming in population, thanks to increased trade with Mexico. What's more, McAllen collected $36 million in Medicaid disproportionate share funding in 1992. That amount was cut in half in 1993 and dropped to about $12 million in 1994. Nonetheless, the border region has been so profitable that Universal recently bought another hospital in the McAllen area, one of the fastest growing metropolitan areas in the country. It's also a booming area for snowbirds—northern tourists who want to escape the cold temperatures. McAllen residents have an old saying that winter Texans arrive just in time to have a heart attack.

Universal also is investing heavily in the Las Vegas market, a demographic gold mine for other investor-owned chains. The company has one hospital there and plans to build two more for a total investment of $90 million.

CHAMPION HEALTHCARE CORPORATION

In May 1989, Paul Queally, a 26-year-old banker at a New York venture capital firm, made a cold call on Charlie Miller. "I want to be your equity partner," Queally said. "I've heard great things about you."

Miller responded that the prospect sounded nice, but he didn't need an equity partner. He had secured bank financing, so there was no need to draw venture capital from Queally's company, the Sprout Group (a division of Donaldson Lufkin & Jenrette). Five months later, Queally came back. "I still want to be your partner," he persisted. Finally, Miller gave in. In 1993, Sprout and a group of other venture capital companies invested $91 million in Champion, which some regard as an early version of Columbia.

Trying to build networks market by market, Champion emanates from a core group of former Republic Health executives. Miller, as noted earlier in the book, was the man who turned down Richard Rainwater's offer to build a hospital company, a turn of events that led to Scott and Rainwater forming Columbia.

Until early 1994, Champion owned only a handful of hospitals in Texas and North Dakota. However, the year brought a burst of acquisitions and a merger with AmeriHealth, a small and financially struggling hospital chain. AmeriHealth's stock was traded on the American Stock Exchange. The merger gave Miller a quick and fairly inexpensive route to becoming a publicly traded company— a strategy Rick Scott also took when he merged Columbia with Smith Labs.

In addition to the merger with AmeriHealth, Champion has since bought a hospital in Salt Lake City from Columbia.

PARACELSUS HEALTHCARE CORPORATION

One of the least-known hospital chains is Paracelsus Healthcare Corporation (Paracelsus). The chain's stock is not publicly traded, but it issued $75 million in publicly traded bonds in 1993. The documents filed in conjunction with that offering provide a small glimpse into a company with more than $400 million in U.S. revenues.

German physician Hartmut Krukemeyer started Paracelsus when he bought the hospital subsidiary of the hotel corporation, Ramada Inns, in 1981. Krukemeyer remained sole owner until his death in May 1994 in Osnabruck, Germany. His son, Manfred George Krukemeyer, inherited the business and became the new owner.

Paracelsus owns hospitals in the United States, Germany, Austria, England, Switzerland, and France, with more than 8,000 beds. U.S. operations of 18 hospitals are handled out of Pasadena, California, by president and CEO R.J. Messenger. About half of the company's hospitals are located in the Los Angeles area. Messenger joined Paracelsus in 1984 after a stint with NME.

DYNAMIC HEALTH

Started by former AMI executive John Silver Jr., Tampa, Florida-based Dynamic owned three hospitals and had a deal to buy two more in early 1995. Silver received venture capital backing from Continental Equity Capital Corporation and Shamrock Investments, Los Angeles, to form Dynamic. The company's hospitals are in rural or suburban markets in Texas, Louisiana, and South Carolina.

The company's first deal was 99-bed River West Medical Center in Plaquemine, Louisiana. Silver worked with a REIT, Healthcare Property Investors, to buy the hospital for $11.5 million then lease it back. Silver left as AMI's chief operating officer in 1990.

Chapter 6

The Abstractions of Finance, Shareholder Value, and Growth

Without money, nothing gets done in this business. That's a blinding flash of the obvious, yet, stressing the monetary side—revenues and profits—doesn't sit well with many healthcare professionals. Perhaps that's one reason why investor-owned chains are often cast as the bad guys in the hospital industry. Their concentration (almost an obsession sometimes) is on revenues and profits.

Ideally, hospitals are supposed to be caring organizations, unaffected by the whims of finance. In reality, the two dynamics (caring and cash flow) must co-exist in the halls of both investor-owned and tax-exempt hospitals. As any tax-exempt hospital executive understands: no profit, no mission.

What makes investor-owned hospitals different isn't necessarily the profit motive. More likely, it's the shareholder motive. These hospital chains operate in a universe controlled by stockholders, a fact that hasn't changed since the birth of AMI, HCA, and Humana.

What has changed since that time is the sheer dollar volume generated by this industry. The healthcare industry (specifically hospitals) has grown from millions to billions, and the magnitude of this enormous cash flow creates opportunities as well as hazards.

"As long as you have an industry that's a multibillion dollar one, people will sit up late at night trying to figure out how to abuse the system in the morning," said Texas State Senator Mike Moncrief, who crusaded against investor-owned psychiatric hospitals during the 1990s. Moncrief vowed: "As long as they stay up, I will also."

Some feel that even though the profit motive is what drives the capitalistic system that America thrives on, it must be uniquely tempered in healthcare.

When HCA founder, Dr. Thomas Frist Sr., joined with six other physicians to build a hospital—actually it started out as a nursing home and was quickly converted to a hospital—he believed the investment aspect would guarantee a high-quality facility.

"All history of business has shown that when people invest their own hard-earned money in any venture, they are on top of it and expect and demand that their money be used in the most efficient, effective, and expeditious manner as possible," Frist declared to the Tennessee Proprietary Hospital Association shortly after founding HCA in 1967. He added, "Those operating such an institution naturally do this better under these circumstances than when they are operating under large grants of money, be they government, church or privately sponsored grants. It's just the nature of the beast."

Yet, this tenet is often skewed in today's cutthroat financial markets. Today's hospital investors do not necessarily operate them; they don't roam the fluorescent-lit halls of their hospitals to ensure that nurses are delivering the best, most efficient care. They're not checking on the mix of tests and drugs and professional skills that determine a patient's care plan.

Rather, today's investors (in healthcare) are mutual fund managers and working families. In most cases, they are simply in pursuit of profit maximization. In Frist's day, if the hospitals he and his partners owned were doing poorly, they would simply work harder to ensure a turnaround. Most of today's investors are more likely to bail out, sell their shares and flock to something else their brokers are hawking, such as Intel Corporation or Viacom.

For the most part, today's hospital company investors are emotionally, geographically, and intellectually distanced from their investment. Among investor-owned hospitals, the financing efforts that take place on a higher level make the corporate assets they hold (namely hospitals) seem transitory. The men and women who know how to push the envelope and keep reaching into the financial bag of tricks are the individuals who soar in this business.

A case in point: By 1993, three of the top four hospital companies had fallen out of favor with Wall Street. NME was mired in government fraud investigations flowing out of its psychiatric hospitals. Humana was struggling with its insurance business. AMI labored under a massive post-LBO debt load. There wasn't anything wrong with the hospital business. In fact, the hospital business almost seems secondary to everything else. Those companies couldn't blame their problems on the hospital business. Arguably, their problems resulted from management missteps.

Today's corporate hospital leaders must be wizards of capital accumulation and allocation. They'll grab a REIT (real estate investment trust), an ESOP (employee stock ownership plan), a junk bond deal, an equity offering, a bank line of credit.

Often investment-owned firms start out with the junk bonds; then sell stock to repay the bonds; then get a bank loan to finance acquisitions, or sell some of the hospitals to a REIT or maybe an ESOP. If the stock price slips, it's probably time for a stock buyback to bolster shareholder confidence. Or, maybe it's time to sell a couple more properties to the REIT or divest some hospitals to raise cash. "Wait a minute, that could stifle earnings. Better look for a couple of acquisitions to pump up the next quarter's figures. How's that debt to capitalization ratio?" Just make sure that stock price keeps rising, quarter after quarter, year after year.

To ensure that ascent (of the stock price) happens, boards often tie a company's stock price to how much they pay the top executives. They want top executives to "feel the pain" of shareholders, as President Bill Clinton would say. If the stock price goes up, the executives are rewarded, usually through stock options. However, this can be a double-edged sword. It grates many middle-class Americans when executives become mega-millionaires by awarding themselves stock, and the feeling is exacerbated when the executives work in the perceptually altruistic field of healthcare.

Perhaps the most striking example of this latter dynamic occurred with Dr. Thomas Frist, Jr., who made $127 million in 1992 after HCA went public for the second time. Frist made that sum because of stock options that he and other HCA executives received when the company went private in 1989. Only $1 million of his 1992 compensation was in salary and bonus—the remainder was realized through the magic of Wall Street.

Such is the risk and reward equation familiar to all entrepreneurs. When Frist took the company private, he put up his entire net worth to get the $4 billion in loans needed. Frist and his family had invested $33 million in HCA when it went private. A loss would have wiped him out. Instead, he hit it big. Rick Scott, founder of Columbia/HCA Healthcare Corporation, also accumulated great wealth through Wall Street's appreciation of his company's stock. Although plenty of investor-owned executives risked little or none of their own money in their companies, both Scott and Frist put their own capital on the line for their companies.

When Republic Health Corporation (now called OrNda Health Corporation) hired Charles Martin to be chairman, president, and CEO in January 1992, Martin bought 1 million shares of the company for $7.75 million to align his interests with those of his new employer.

ALIGNING PHYSICIANS THROUGH FINANCIAL INCENTIVES

If it makes sense to ensure that top executives own stock in the company, wouldn't it also make sense to make customers equity holders? That is precisely the logic behind Columbia's strategy of physician ownership, as mentioned earlier in the book. Physicians control nearly every aspect of a patient's care. Without them, a hospital wouldn't have any business.

However, tying physicians' financial interests with those of the hospital is a complex process and a legal minefield. Columbia believes it has structured its deals with physicians in the most appropriate legal manner. It's important to note that patient referrals do not affect the return on investment of physicians in Columbia hospitals. That would run afoul of federal fraud and abuse laws.

Physician owners who invest in Columbia are compensated based on the amount of their investment, not the amount of business they bring in the doors.

Despite Columbia's reliance on this strategy, it hasn't been widely imitated among its peers. Republic began doing joint ventures with physicians on all of its hospitals for a while. However, when Martin was hired as new president and CEO, he stopped that process and dissolved the physician joint ventures that were in place. "I don't think the most efficient way to tie the physicians today is to sell them a piece of the production side—the hospital," Martin said.

Rick Scott apparently feels otherwise. Columbia has syndicated healthcare networks in El Paso, Fort Lauderdale, San Antonio, and Orlando.

One important feature of these offerings was that doctors couldn't invest in Columbia's network and a competing network. In fact, the document stipulated that an investor couldn't invest in an acute-care hospital, specialty hospital, rehab facility, outpatient center, or other ambulatory venture. Such a proviso prevented Columbia's doctors from opening a surgery center across the street—an event that has happened to more than one hospital and actually happened frequently to Humana hospitals.

Medical Care America, a Dallas-based outpatient surgery center company fed on the needs of disgruntled doctors. It opened several surgery centers across the street from Humana hospitals. How was it able to accomplish such a tactic? Fundamentally, Humana had upset its doctors with the Humana Care Plus health plan, which scrutinized their admissions and in some cases capitated their payments. Humana and its physicians became enemies in a handful of cities, and to "exact revenge," some of those doctors took their surgery business elsewhere.

In 1994, Columbia bought Medical Care America. One reason the deal fit so well was that Columbia had acquired all of the former Humana hospitals.

Preventing doctors from investing in competing healthcare businesses didn't last long for Columbia, though. The company was later forced by the state of Florida to drop the noncompete clause in its syndications. Still, critics question whether physicians who invest will let their pocketbook dictate medical decisions.

FAVORABLE FINANCING: SUPREME RESULTS

Interestingly, physician equity can make a big difference. Witness San Antonio. Humana had four hospitals there that lost a combined $40 million in 1992 because of horrible relations with their physicians.

One of the hospital's CEOs, Earl Denning, left in 1992, claiming that relations got so bad, physicians had "spit on and verbally abused" him. After Columbia announced the merger with Galen (the Humana hospital spin-off) in mid-1993, he came back.

"The doctors are beginning to look at the hospital in a new light," Denning said. Since returning to Galen's San Antonio Regional Hospital, Denning met with four or five doctors a day and found them "phenomenally positive" about the future and the merger with Columbia. About 125 of them also bought into Columbia's San Antonio network.

Getting executives and physicians to invest in a hospital company gives them a sense of control. But let's look at this another way. Because of the way the stock market works, the tables may turn. Instead of the executive in charge getting more and more stock, a stockholder may accumulate enough stock to take charge. In publicly held companies, majority rules; and once the majority shifts, the rules may change drastically.

A classic example of this process was provided by Republic Health Corporation. Dallas-based Republic was founded by a handful of former Hospital Affiliates executives who bought 18 hospitals from HCA. By 1983, Republic was ready to go public and succeeded with a fruitful public offering, thanks to its then-attorney Rick Scott.

Going public made Republic executives eager for the type of growth needed to fuel the company's stock price. As Republic's share price sagged, the need to expand became even more critical. Fortunately, Republic executives found their avenue for growth in three hospitals owned by Health Resources Corp. of America, a public company whose motto was "The company that's doing well while doing good!"

One of the hospitals, Houston Northwest Medical Center, was a treasure chest. Its EBITDA (earnings before interest, taxes, depreciation, and amortization) alone was $30 million a year—plenty to sustain an entire midsized hospital company. At one point, Houston Northwest would produce 25 percent of Republic's cash flow—a staggering amount for a stable of more than 50 hospitals.

Republic acquired Healthcare Resources in a $93 million stock swap that shifted the balance of power to Healthcare's founder, LeRoy A. Pesch M.D. With the acquisition, Pesch became Republic's single largest shareholder.

Pesch was well-versed in the hospital business. He had been quoted prominently in an October 26, 1974, *Business Week* article, "Why the nation's hospitals may well go broke." As president of Chicago's highly regarded Michael Reese Hospital and Medical

Center, Pesch said, "Clearly the financial pressures on hospitals have to be resolved if the institutions as we know them today are going to survive."

Based on that prognostication, it might seem odd that Pesch would dive into the hospital business. Yet he did, starting Healthcare Resources with $40 million in funding from his father-in-law and Chicago insurance magnate W. Clement Stone. When Republic bought Pesch's hospitals, the company also gave him a board seat, a common trade-off for significant shareholders.

In late 1985, new Republic director Pesch came up with a plan to take the company private and convinced CEO James Buncher and CFO James McAtee to go along. He gathered financial support from Wall Street's junk bond generator, Drexel Burnham Lambert.

After some fussing on price, the LBO was done in August 1986, and in February 1987 Pesch scampered off to conquer another buyout target, American Medical International. Fresh from the Republic deal—in which bankers and bond dealers split $33 million in fees —Pesch believed he could gather support to do it all over again. He didn't. AMI turned him down and thus dodged a bullet.

Meanwhile, Pesch's Republic began spinning into a deep financial spiral under the weight of $850 million in LBO debt. In its first year as a private company, Republic lost $283 million. The company soon was forced to bring turnaround consultants Alvarez & Marsal from New York. Brian Marsal was named the company's CEO although he had never run a hospital company before.

The long journey back was painful and expensive. Alvarez & Marsal would be paid more than $5 million in fees from 1990 to 1992. The surviving corporation, renamed OrNda HealthCorp, is barely recognizable as the old Republic.

Republic's experience shows, however, that daredevil acrobatics on a financial high-wire act can be a precipitous route to a hospital company's decline. As Marsal proved at Republic, executives with no hospital experience are sometimes hired to right the ship once its finances have gone astray. One current example is NME's chairman, president and CEO Jeffrey Barbakow, whose experience formerly was in investment banking and the entertainment industry.

Another example occurred in 1988 when AMI's revolving door of leadership appeared to open briefly to Morton Meyerson, an AMI board member and former president of Electronic Data Systems. Ira

Korman, who was running one of the most profitable Humana hospitals in the country, Medical City Dallas, recalls an incident in which he was having a casual meeting with Rick Scott, then just starting the fledgling Columbia Hospital Corporation. At that time, Scott was still working out of the offices of his partner, Richard Rainwater. After a short tour of the office, Scott suggested that Korman meet Rainwater. Korman remembered that Rainwater went into a tirade about the industry's big four—AMI, NME, HCA, and Humana. Those companies wouldn't exist if they had to start over today, Rainwater said. The only reason they've survived is that they had a 25-year jump.

"Actually, it turned out to be prophetic," Korman said. "Because after that everything started to unravel." Within four years of that meeting, all four companies would be restructuring for a variety of reasons.

However, it's what Rainwater said next that Korman recalls best. Rainwater was part of a group that owned a large interest in AMI, and he told Korman that AMI's board was considering Meyerson for the post of CEO. "Would Korman come over some afternoon and teach Meyerson about the hospital business?" Rainwater asked. Korman was incredulous. "An afternoon?"

Meyerson, for reasons that were never publicized, wasn't hired. If he had been, it would be easy to guess the first words out of his mouth: *shareholder value*. In other words, get the stock price up. Some hospital chain executives carry beepers so they can be reached, but the beepers also enable them to check their company's stock price instantly.

KEEPING SHAREHOLDERS LOYAL

"The number one priority for our board is to drive shareholder value," President and CEO Jeffrey Barbakow said in a conference call with analysts when he announced National Medical Enterprises' $3.1 billion acquisition of American Medical International in late 1994. Whenever a public company gets in trouble, the first thing out of the CEO's mouth is a vow to maximize shareholder value. Get the stock price up.

If a company's stock price falls, it will mar the ability to complete mergers, make acquisitions, recruit talented professionals, even secure bank financing. If the stock price plunges, there may be no end to the trouble.

When a company gets into financial problems, a series of events typically happen. Each is like a block being pulled out in the popular game of Jenga. Eventually, if more and more blocks are pulled, the stack will fall. Usually, these events start with a quarterly earnings report. A company finds out its numbers are not going to be as high as expected. The CEO or CFO calls the company's investment banker, usually the one who did an equity or bond offering for the company, to warn them to adjust earnings forecasts.

If the numbers are very poor, the company could be in default of its bank credit agreements. It wouldn't have to miss a payment to do that; it could just be out of certain financial "ratios" for debt, profits, or cash. If the stock price falls too much, lawsuits by the shareholders are sure to follow, especially if the stock falls suddenly after a poor earnings announcement or other bad news. Sometimes, a company's stock falls if quarterly earning don't meet analysts' estimates. In other words, the company made more money but not as much as predicted.

Basically, two types of companies are attractive to investors: growth companies and value companies. Growth companies trade at a high price/earnings (p/e) ratio that is synonymous to their growth rate. Simply put, a p/e ratio of 50 means investors expect this company to grow at a 50 percent annual rate, a pretty remarkable clip.

Value companies are those that aren't making great expansion strides, but they're safe and strong. Investors can expect their money to grow somewhat—maybe not double in a year, but outpace bank certificates of deposit (CDs) or Treasury bonds.

At some point, the lines must merge. A growth company will become a value company. As short sellers say, trees don't grow to the sky. Growth in a mature company won't be able to maintain the same growth rate as a start-up. Start-up operations may not attract much attention initially on Wall Street, but once they get going, a start-up company can soon become a cash-rich machine, throwing off fees with every bond, equity, and merger deal in its path.

When an investment bank collects huge fees for underwriting a bond or stock deal, it often promises research support. That means that its research analysts will issue reports on the company's stock. Although a positive report isn't necessarily promised, it's often given.

For example, Healthtrust did a widely successful initial public offering in December 1991 that raised more than $500 million. Since its spin-off in 1987, the company's CEO, R. Clayton McWhorter, knew he must head in one direction, taking the company public. It was the only way that Healthtrust could generate enough cash to buy back HCA's preferred stock. Merrill Lynch, a New York-based investment banker, was named as lead underwriter for the Healthtrust offering and promptly began to line up investors to buy the stock.

Before and immediately after going public, a company and its underwriters go through a "quiet period" in which they cannot promote the stock. This is a standard requirement enforced by the Securities and Exchange Commission.

On January 9, 1992, the quiet period expired on Healthtrust. That same day, Merrill's healthcare analyst, Lucy Olwell, put out a "buy" rating on Healthtrust shares, saying they were "extremely underpriced." The stock soared. In one day, it rose 20 percent, with 4.5 million shares trading hands.

Investors had already been richly rewarded. Thanks to that extra punch, Healthtrust shares had appreciated 60 percent since the offering in December. What a return for investors; what a coup for underwriter Merrill Lynch.

Investment bankers can make an ugly duckling look like a beautiful swan—if it suits them financially. Even Columbia made that transformation. Initially, Wall Street shunned the company. In a December 4, 1992, profile of Columbia, inveterate Dillon Read analyst Carl Sherman warned about Columbia's tendency to purchase financially troubled hospitals, "Anytime you buy distressed merchandise, you're at risk," cautioned Sherman.

However, after Columbia pulled off the Galen and HCA mergers, the feeling on Wall Street changed. Eager for the generous fees associated with merger and acquisition activity, and equity and bond sales, New York investment banking firms lusted for Columbia's business. Scott did not disappoint. He soon acquired a knack for spreading the business around, not staying with any one investment banking firm for all of the company's business. Donaldson, Lufkin & Jenrette; Morgan Stanley & Co.; Merrill Lynch & Co.; Dillon, Read & Co.; Kidder, Peabody & Co.; Smith Barney, Harris Upham & Co.—all have had their names on the lower third of a Columbia equity or offering.

By spreading the wealth around, Columbia received another round of support from stock analysts.

RURAL VERSUS NONURBAN HOSPITALS

Wall Street can be fickle, however. One case in point lies in rural hospitals. Because of the previous debacles by National Healthcare, Westworld, and Gateway Medical (mentioned in earlier chapters), Wall Street shied away from rural hospital chains. However, rural hospital chains didn't go by the wayside; they just changed their stripes. They became "nonurban" hospital chains.

When Health Management Associates went public at $10 a share in 1986, the first sentence of the company's prospectus said the hospital chain provided "a broad range of general acute-care health services to rural communities." After doing a leveraged buyout in 1988, HMA went public again in 1991. This time the first sentence of the prospectus said the company provided "a broad range of general acute care health services in non-urban communities." Not much had changed, just the lingo.

Yet, HMA is a good example of the fickle swings of Wall Street. Wall Street initially treated HMA pretty poorly, lumping them in with other rural hospitals chains that had historically treated Wall Street pretty poorly. Analysts preferred to recommend the more cosmopolitan chains, such as Humana, National Medical Enterprises, and American Medical International. Although HMA logged consistent profits, the company's stock never traded above its $10 per share offering price until mid-1988, and then it was only in the $11 range.

"It's in a bad industry," healthcare analyst Paul Szczgiel at Bear Sterns explained at the time. "They did a stellar job, but everybody kept wondering when something might break." So, Schoen and his

venture capital colleagues decided to take the company off the
public market through an LBO.

Even though hospital chains like Republic Health Corp. and
Charter Medical Corp. were nearly strangled by the LBO debt they
took on, HMA chugged along, business as usual. When the company went public again in February 1991, Wall Street was agog. The
shares originally were priced at $13.50, but demand was so great
that the price increased to $16.

"There's nothing different about the company," Schoen acknowledged at the time when asked about the contrast in the company's
demand from investors. For Schoen and his backers, the deal was
wildly profitable. First Chicago and Prudential Venture Capital
Management came away with a 400 percent profit in just a little over
two years. Both had kicked in $9.25 million to help fund the buyout
in 1988. At the offering price, the stakes were now worth $51 million
each.

Since that time, HMA has continued to move along without
stumbling. The hospital chain has few detractors and has managed
to retain one of the cleanest reputations in the industry. Thanks to
HMA and Healthtrust, investment bankers began saying good things
about rural hospitals. In a March 1993 research report, J.P. Morgan
& Co. reported that Healthtrust's rural hospitals were an asset
because they "may be particularly well protected from any adverse
impact of healthcare reform." There was ample evidence for opti-
mism. Even though Healthtrust still carried a heavy debt load, its
margins were great. The company had an EBITDA margin of 21
percent, higher than many of its competitors.

IF STOCKS TURN SOUR...

What happens if hospitals fall out of favor on Wall Street, and the
stock market leaves Columbia in the dust? Won't the company
break up just like HCA did in the late 1980s? McWhorter—formerly
with Healthtrust and now with Columbia—thinks not, relying on
what experience has taught him.

"It didn't work in 1987," he says. It's true. Spinning off Healthtrust
didn't help HCA's stock price.

As Columbia grew, it became a more attractive investment vehicle. It financed the big acquisitions—Galen, HCA, and Healthtrust—through stock swaps, which didn't dilute shareholder value or add debt. In fact, when Columbia merged with HCA, stock analysts loved it because it meant Columbia's debt-to-equity ratio would drop from 53 percent to 45 percent. Debt-to-equity ratios measure the amount of funds owed to creditors with the amount of assets supplied by owners.

Across the board, the national average for debt to equity is about 33 percent, but hospital companies typically run higher because the business has high capital needs and tends to be higher leveraged to finance those needs.

Maybe Wall Street doesn't like the spin-offs, but it loves the consolidations. They see potential in the work of the 1990s hospital consolidators. For example, in the Columbia merger with Healthtrust, the estimated savings break down is as follows:

- $5 million in overhead
- $5 million in data processing
- $75 million in purchasing
- $10 million in interest costs
- $5 million in local market consolidation
- $25 million in fringe benefit programs.

Not coincidentally, Columbia is squeezing vendors for bigger discounts at a time when the suppliers are scrambling for business. A classic illustration used in the healthcare industry is that when costs are squeezed out of one area, they balloon in another. For example, when Medicare imposed diagnostic related groups (DRGs) on the inpatient side of the business, the outpatient side mushroomed.

Profits for hospital management companies in the early 1990s came at the expense of medical supply and technology vendors. Hit by falling profits, the stock prices of those vendors in 1994 reflected the turmoil in that industry, buffeted by cost-containment and threats of health reform. Hospital supplier companies saw their stock prices drop 3 percent in 1994 and drug makers' stock prices dropped 22 percent. Not surprisingly, suppliers were willing to make concessions in exchange for guaranteed volume from the biggest powerhouse in the industry, Columbia/HCA.

The irony of the consolidations that led to Columbia's size isn't lost on industry old-timers, however. "You tear the old down so it will work better and then you put it back together so it will work better," says OrNda chairman Charles Martin. In other words, HCA spun off Healthtrust so both companies could focus on their own hospitals, and now Columbia has put them back together.

Yet, growth for the sake of growth can be a menace. In the early 1990s, National Medical Enterprises became mired in problems because of its psychiatric hospital operations. After a wide-ranging investigation that included federal agents storming the company's Santa Monica headquarters, the company paid a record $379 million fine to settle massive federal fraud charges.

How did a hospital company get in such trouble? NME's co-founder John Bedrosian fingered the culprit as too much growth. "The driving force has been to grow, grow, grow," he testified in January 1992 before a Texas legislative committee investigating abuses among psychiatric hospitals.

State Senator Moncrief asked, "Growth for growth sake or growth for profit sake?" Bedrosian answered, "The same thing, senator." Further pressed, Bedrosian said the pressure to grow drove some of its employees to [engage] in overly aggressive and unethical practices because they placed profits too high on their list of priorities.

When NME was founded, Bedrosian and his two cofounders, Richard Eamer and Leonard Cohen, would go to every board meeting of the hospitals they owned. But that fell by the wayside as the company got bigger and bigger. Soon, corporate management was detached from hospital management.

Bedrosian added, "Very candidly, in Los Angeles, we did not know what was going on in Texas. PIA (Psychiatric Institutes of America, NME's psych subsidiary) had done well for years and so we simply said 'God bless you. Keep going.'" Then, he blamed the subsidiary's problems on "one individual or two, who are no longer with the company and haven't been for many months."

Yet, in a later deposition, Bedrosian seems to have shown little interest in altering his detached style. At the hearing before the Texas legislative committee, Bedrosian relates how he flew into

Austin on NME's corporate jet, showed up at the hearing, testified for 15 minutes, then left.

At the deposition, Bedrosian was asked, "Did you ask anybody in Texas, 'Say, what are they talking about when they're accusing us of indulging in headhunting fees and bounties?'"

Bedrosian: "No, sir, I did not."

Attorney: "You did not."

Bedrosian: "I never had an opportunity."

In his deposition, Bedrosian said he also hadn't reviewed patient files that were the subject of lawsuits. "I have had our operating people just tell me generically that these people are making allegations that are not well-founded, that we have good records and files on these people, and that...we are unable to disclose any of that material because of confidentiality laws; and therefore, we were being shellacked in the press without an opportunity to be heard."

Yes, but how did the shareholders make out?

SOMETIMES SHAREHOLDERS LOSE BIG

Devotion to shareholder value only goes so far, however, when investor-owned companies set up complex financing strategies. If the business goes into bankruptcy reorganization, who's at the bottom of the creditor list? Shareholders. The government gets its money first. For example, if a financially distressed company has an outstanding claims with the IRS, the feds take their money off the top.

As senior lenders, banks typically will get their money next. Next on the creditor list are bondholders and a variety of others to whom the company owes money. The very last name on the list is the shareholder, who may get nothing.

An example of this took place with Healthcare International, an Austin, Texas-based chain that owned 15 psychiatric and four acute-care hospitals when it began running into trouble in 1989. Healthcare International filed for bankruptcy reorganization, in November 1991. As part of the reorganization, Healthcare International merged into the owner of most of its properties, a real estate investment trust called HealthVest.

HealthVest shareholders got 96 percent of the equity in the new company, called Healthcare America; bondholders got the remaining 4 percent and Healthcare International shareholders got nothing.

How the mighty had fallen. Healthcare International initially prospered by building plush mental health hospitals that won architecture awards. These lush structures featured such country-club amenities as gymnasiums, amphitheaters, swimming pools, music rooms, and open-air dining pavilions. No expense was spared. To generate cash, Healthcare International went public in October 1985. However, its executives were disappointed with the amount of capital raised—just $20 million, hardly enough to finance an aggressive expansion. The timing had been bad—the offering came right after HCA announced a drop in profits, making investors nervous about a new hospital company.

So, the company's executives launched a REIT, HealthVest, in June 1986 that raised $112 million. It was so successful that they sold more stock in March 1987, raising another $112 million. The REIT also borrowed $150 million from a group of six banks. The money just kept coming.

By way of background, REITs are usually publicly traded corporations that specialize in purchasing and managing real estate properties. They were created to buy such tame properties as shopping centers and office buildings. Dealing with a REIT is kind of like dealing with a bank. You borrow money, and you work out a repayment schedule.

Here's how it works. As a REIT, you own properties. You collect rent. You take out expenses—which are the amortized cost of the properties—and figure out what your profit is. REITs generally do not pay state or federal taxes, so nearly all of the profit is distributed in dividends to shareholders. In the mid-1980s, the hospital industry was going through financial turmoil, and they saw some easy money here. Soon, National Medical Enterprises, American Medical International, and Universal Health Services were all starting REITs. Healthcare International, however, really pushed the financial envelope on its REIT. As a result, the hospital company's shareholders came out on the short end.

The most crucial decisions a REIT manager has to make, obviously, are what properties to buy and for how much. If you already own and operate those properties, would that cloud your vision on those decisions? It did at HealthVest, which paid too much for the hospitals it bought. That led to the financial downfall of the REIT. And, it also put the hospital company into bankruptcy because Healthcare International ended up with rental and mortgage payments that were more than the hospitals were worth.

Ironically, investors in the REIT were getting less than those in the hospital company—they were just getting the real estate. However, at that time Wall Street liked the real estate business better than the hospital business, so it got a higher valuation.

Unfortunately, HealthVest, the REIT, depended on the hospital company for 93 percent of its revenues. Both companies shared the same managers even though they answered to separate groups of shareholders. As a means of raising capital, the REIT worked. It funneled more than $400 million to Healthcare International. However, eventually too many investors owned pieces of too few assets. In addition to the money raised from the equity offerings, HealthVest had borrowed some $200 million from banks. Healthcare International—the hospitals' operator—had sold junk bonds as well. That meant that banks, the bondholders, and the shareholders of the two companies all laid claim to the same group of hospitals.

If the hospitals continue to produce profits, great! But if they don't, there will be two, not one, group of stockholders who are upset. What's more, a REIT complicates the financial structure of the company, prompting more lawyers and accountants to get involved, and that means more expense. "At some point, it all catches up with you," said Robertson Colman & Stephens analyst Jerry Balter in 1989.

In April 1989, HealthVest president Elliott H. Weir Jr., who was also executive vice president of Healthcare International, predicted boom times ahead for the REIT. "We...are confident that the year will continue to reflect the growth trends established over the past three years," he said. Oops. HealthVest ended the year with a loss of $116.8 million, and banks poised to foreclose.

Healthcare International had sold its hospitals at a top-dollar price to the REIT. Now, it was having problems generating enough cash to pay its monthly notes to the REIT. That put the REIT in financial trouble as well. Healthcare International went into a bankruptcy reorganization in which the only ones who came out ahead were the banks. The company's $217 million in loans remained due.

Only a year out of bankruptcy reorganization, Healthcare America—with 12 hospitals in six states—began choking on its bank loans again in 1995. Those hospitals continue to grapple with a way of financially balancing their revenues and expenses.

Hospital companies aren't alone in shafting shareholders when money troubles arrive. Obviously, investors have lost money in all kinds of companies. However, it shows the complex financial dilemmas hospitals can get themselves into when they choose to become for-profit. A tax-exempt hospital traditionally uses tax-exempt debt to finance expansions or renovations because that's the cheapest money available.

While the hospital must, in theory, answer to bondholders, it likely won't develop the complex web of financiers of an investor-owned hospital. As we said before, investor-owned hospitals are different not because they must make a profit, but because they answer to shareholders. Yet, it almost never ends at shareholders.

Almost without exception, investor-owned companies develop another whole genus of money masters: junk bondholders, banks, venture capital investors, private placement investors, and real estate investment trusts.

REITS LIVE ON

Despite the drastic example of Healthcare International and HealthVest, REITs remain popular although none are as dependent on a single hospital company as HealthVest was on Healthcare International.

In fact, REITS are more widespread than ever because they offer investors a high rate of return that is viewed as safe. Between fall 1992 and spring 1994, REITs raised more than $15 billion in new equity and convertible securities, according to Natwest Securities. Only 10 percent of that money went to healthcare REITs, however.

Healthcare REITs offer high dividends, portfolio growth, and capital appreciation potential, according to a March 1994 report from NatWest Securities, a New York-based investment banking firm that specializes in healthcare REITS.

In 1993, the average total return of the typical healthcare REIT was 22 percent, compared with 10 percent total return for the Standard & Poor's 500, according to NatWest.

There are nine healthcare REITs, although about half of them handle only long-term-care properties. The average REIT has a market capitalization of about $400 million, according to NatWest.

One of the newest and most active healthcare REITs is Healthcare Realty Trust, a Nashville-based firm started by David Emery. Columbia is one of Healthcare's biggest customers, but not for its hospitals. Columbia has sold its outpatient and medical office buildings to the REIT, then leased them back. Some not-for-profit hospitals have also turned to REITs for funding, but most have not needed to. Tax-exempt bonds cost far less, with interest rates at least 2 percentage points below the 10 or 11 percent financing offered by a REIT. Even so, REITs provide a flexibility to for-profits that not-for-profits may lack.

For example, when Healthtrust was having trouble getting financing for a new hospital in Austin, Texas, National Health Investors agreed to put up the $86 million. Another REIT, American Health Properties, asked to join the deal and took a $30 million participation in the loan. By the way, half of American Health's revenues come from six hospitals owned by American Medical International, which started the REIT in 1987. The largest healthcare REIT is Meditrust, with $1.3 billion in assets. It has completed seven equity offerings since 1985. REITs are simply another way to buy, sell, and trade hospitals.

A HEALTHCARE COMMODITY TO BUY AND SELL

Hospitals—where surgeons delicately repair damaged hearts, and machines pump small puffs of air into underweight babies—become like just so many chocolates in a box. Let's move the creamy caramel one from this box to that box. From a county hospital authority to Health Management Associates. From Quorum Health Group to Columbia.

Here are places where life and death dance together amidst anxious families and skilled practitioners. Yet, as hospitals are passed back and forth like children of divorced parents, one might wonder, Doesn't it matter who owns these institutions? Perhaps not. The leaders of investor-owned hospital companies aren't managing hospitals as much as they're managing money. They hire people to manage the hospitals, but their first priority is managing the money properly.

Consider this. When Columbia merged with HCA in 1994, Rick Scott essentially took over a company that had been owned, at least in part, by the Frist family since its founding. Either Thomas Frist, Jr., or Sr. had always headed that company. Now, Frist Jr. was turning over day-to-day operations to Scott. This was not a decision Frist could take lightly. His family's stake in HCA was valued at $690 million.

In simple terms, he was turning that investment over to Scott to manage. He trusted Scott to be the best manager of that fortune. Scott's track record was indeed impressive. Although Frist had made $120 million on his stock when HCA went public again, HCA shares hadn't appreciated much since the offering. During the same period, Columbia shares had doubled. Obviously, Frist made the right choice in turning his fortune over to Scott's command. Columbia's merger deal with HCA lifted HCA shares 40 percent.

Leaders like Scott and Frist manage hospital chains, but most of all they manage investors. Their fate will be decided by how well they manage the equity portion of their balance sheet.

MORE NOT-FOR-PROFIT HOSPITALS TURN TO INVESTOR-OWNED CHAINS

Why would a hospital, after collecting years of goodwill equity in a community, want to become another cog in the corporate machinery? Often the driving factor is money, or lack thereof.

Sometimes the hospital is losing money, or maybe the hospital's board is afraid that their hospital will start losing money if it doesn't merge with a larger system.

Of course, the reasons given rarely mention money as the instigator. For example, consider a recent alignment in Denver. "We will be able to develop a truly integrated system as we continue to provide high-quality, cost-effective healthcare for our community," stated Stephen Kurtz, chairman of Rose Healthcare System (Rose), in announcing its pending sale to Columbia/HCA Healthcare Corporation in 1995.

Kurtz's accounting firm, Shenkin Kurtz Baker & Co., then turned around and issued a press release noting that the hospital board chairman had "put together the recent sale of Denver's Rose Healthcare System." The juxtaposition of the two events was described in the *Denver Post* as "unabashed self-promotion" on the part of Kurtz. Even so, Kurtz's hands-on experience in the Rose deal will probably be good for his business.

Correspondingly, Columbia's acquisition of Rose in the competitive Denver market will be good for its business. No doubt, the Rose Healthcare System assimiliation into Columbia's three-hospital Denver area system will be good for Rose's business.

Rose was one of dozens of tax-exempt hospitals that received buyout offers amid a virtual feeding frenzy in 1993 and 1994. Sellers have the incentive to become part of a network in a quickly consolidating market. Buyers have the incentive to grow, a virtue that will lead to a higher valuation from Wall Street. Every Monday morning at 7 A.M., Columbia's Rick Scott has a teleconference with his managers throughout the country. They talk strategy and, most importantly, deals in the works. At an analysts' meeting in September 1994, Columbia's senior vice president Vic Campbell described how the meetings go: "Last Monday, there was a list of 72 of them (potential acquisitions). Two months ago there were 33."

Columbia seems to keep those cards and letters coming in. The incentive to grow reaches to individual employees at investor-owned chains. For example, at Quorum Health Group, a Nashville-based hospital chain, employees were offered $25,000 for sales leads that would give Quorum a jump on Columbia and other acquirers.

"Once the fact that a hospital is considering purchase, joint venture or lease option becomes general knowledge, it's generally too late to make a move," said a Quorum in-house newsletter, adding, "We have to get in there early, that's when we can do some good, so you can see that passing crucial information along quickly is most important."

Once in the door, negotiations can be the most interesting part. In many cases, seasoned mergers and acquisition specialists from investor-owned chains are pitted against hospital trustees who have never before sold a hospital. It's been said that when a man with money meets a man with experience, the man with experience ends up with the money, and the man with money ends up with the experience.

For example, Columbia last year agreed to buy Bishop Clarkson Hospital in Omaha for $85 million. That's not all Bishop Clarkson will receive, though. The hospital has another sugar daddy who will kick in $12 million, namely Uncle Sam. It seems that Bishop Clarkson didn't take enough depreciation when it filed its annual Medicare cost reports. Since the hospital is changing ownership, it must file a "terminating cost report" to financially settle up with the government.

Based on the sale price, Medicare owes the hospital $12 million, a 14 percent premium on top of the $85 million sale price. The $12 million is called "Medicare recapture." In this case, Bishop Clarkson's foundation benefits because it will receive the sale proceeds. However, sometimes, it doesn't work that way, especially if the hospital isn't a savvy negotiator.

"If it [Medicare recapture] is an asset, you try to take it; if it's a liability, you try to give it away," said Joshua Nemzoff, who specializes in mergers and acquisitions for Nashville-based Nemzoff & Co.

For example, if a hospital isn't aware of the Medicare recapture potential, the buyer might offer, "We'll settle up with Medicare for you. You don't want that hassle." Sounds reasonable, considering it sometimes takes a couple of years to finally settle with Medicare. On the other hand, if the hospital is selling for much more than the price at which it's been valued, the seller could end up with a big bill from Medicare. Such a bill would effectively lower the sale price of the hospital.

Another case in point, when Montgomery County Hospital District sold its Conroe, Texas, hospital to Healthtrust in 1993, the district found that it owed $8.5 million in Medicare recapture. Although that sounds grim, there was a happy ending. Ken Thornton, the district's executive director, said, "the county hired experts from two big accounting firms—Price Waterhouse and Deloitte & Touche." And voila! Now Medicare owes the district $1.6 million. The moral to this anecdote is, hire the right accountants and lawyers and the numbers may eventually work in your favor.

Finding the right talent is crucial to this and other processes in the buy/sell transaction. Consider this: Columbia frequently works with three managers in the Miami office of Ernst & Young who do nothing but Medicare recapture work. When millions of dollars are at stake, it pays to call a specialist.

SPEAKING IN EBITDA TERMS

Like visitors to a foreign country, not-for-profit hospital boards and executives need to learn about the "exchange rates" in this new world of mergers and acquisitions. That exchange rate is known as EBITDA. Until the late 1980s, hospital companies typically valued the transaction based on the number of beds. For example, Wesley Medical Center's purchase by HCA was valued at nearly $350,000 a bed—a huge sum.

However, during the late 1980s, Columbia and other companies started talking in terms of EBITDA—earnings before interest, taxes, depreciation, and amortization. That provides a function for value among all hospitals, tax-paying and tax-exempt. EBITDA is a much different figure than asset worth, and one that gives a better snapshot of a hospital's earnings power at the time of sale.

Once the EBITDA is determined, a multiple of the calculation is used to determine a sales price. Generally, the investor-owned chains say they want to pay between six to seven times EBITDA. When Columbia announced the deal for HCA, the multiple was seven times EBITDA, but by the time the transaction actually closed, it had escalated to nearly nine (8.7 to be precise) times EBITDA, according to J.P. Morgan Securities, New York. The multiple rose because Columbia's stock price swelled. A stock swap is based on a ratio (e.g. one share for one and one-half shares), and that ratio likely won't change after the deal is announced. Of course, if one company's stock craters, the deal could be off.

Although hospital chains use six or seven times EBITDA as a guide, that number can vary. Additionally, it depends on whether a buyer is paying a multiple of current EBITDA or future EBITDA. For example, Deborah Moffett, chief financial officer of Community Health Systems (Community), said the Houston-based hospital chain doesn't want to pay more than 4.5 times first-year EBITDA.

A case in point: Community bought Scott County Hospital in Oneida, Tennessee, for 18 times EBITDA, which sounds way out of line. Yet, after the first year under Community's management, profits at the 99-bed hospital soared so much that the sale price amounted to just 1.2 times EBITDA. The same was true in Enid, Oklahoma, where Community bought a hospital at 14.2 times

EBITDA. After the first year, the recalculation amounted to only 2.3 times EBITDA.

Frankly, chains such as Columbia or Community often pay a higher multiple for what might appear to be an average, "run-of-the-mill" not-for-profit hospital than a comparable investor-owned facility. Why the discrepancy? The large systems believe that some of the not-for-profit hospitals are not as well managed and can subsequently become more profitable under their purview.

"You have to look at upside potential," said Earl Holland, who focuses on acquisitions for Health Management Associates, a Naples, Florida-based firm.

Another factor that affects price is how much the investor-owned chain wants the hospital. The price may rise if the hospital is critical to network development and if the bidding is intense. It's not unusual for a hospital to have 15 bidders responding to an offer, known as a request for proposal (RFP).

Once a chain buys a hospital, EBITDA remains an important statistic. For example, when Quorum bought St. Anthony's Medical Center in Columbus, Ohio, in February 1992 for $15 million, the hospital had a slim $1 million of EBITDA. That multiple makes the acquisition look pretty pricey: 15 times EBITDA. However, Quorum turned the hospital around. By 1993, the facility (now called Park Medical Center) reported $7.4 million in EBITDA, and in 1994 that number increased to $9.5 million.

Those are the types of figures Quorum and other investor-owned chains strive to highlight when they talk to Wall Street's investment bankers to show the increasing profitability of their hospitals.

EBITDA is also important in joint ventures with tax-exempt hospitals. For example, when Columbia entered into a 50–50 joint venture in San Antonio with Southwest Texas Methodist Hospital, the value of each partner's share was determined by EBITDA. Methodist's valuation was $255 million; Columbia's four hospitals were valued at $131 million, meaning that Columbia had to put cash into the deal to make up its 50 percent. Through joint ventures with investor-owned chains, tax-exempt hospitals can have their cake and eat it too. They can sell a majority stake in the hospital and retain cash flow—kind of like an annuity that keeps paying an annual dividend.

For example, in New Orleans, Columbia/HCA bought an 80 percent interest in Tulane University Medical Center for $128 million. Tulane gets a huge cash infusion to use for research or fund its endowment, and it still gets 20 percent of the profits in future years.

Columbia's Scott believes this type of deal will appeal to other medical schools that own hospitals. "These schools got into the business to teach medical students," Scott says. "We can help them control costs and ensure that they have access to patients. They can't get that if they're not efficient and not part of a provider network." Teaching hospitals have been notoriously higher priced than other hospitals. As such, they are being excluded from some managed-care plans that don't want to pay the additional expense of teaching medical students.

Columbia has been making a push to buy academic medical centers, but its most significant deal in that area fell apart in 1994. Under pressure from Georgia not-for-profit hospitals and its own medical staff, Emory University's two hospitals broke off a deal with Columbia/HCA.

It would have been difficult to "slam dunk" Columbia's corporate culture into Emory's academic identity, noted Sandra Person Burns, executive director of the Atlanta Healthcare Alliance. Such a deal is "90 percent cultural and 10 percent contractual, but Columbia thought it was 10 percent cultural and 90 percent contractual," she said. Another Georgia hospital, Southern Regional Medical Center in Riverdale, also turned down an offer from Columbia. "The implications were too great," said hospital president Donald P. Logan about the prospect of changing the hospital's status to investor-owned.

FINANCIAL PRESSURES IMPINGE ON DECISION MAKING

Financial pressures are bearing hard on tax-exempt institutions. In 1990, for-profit hospitals had the lowest average margin on prospective payment: negative 4.5 percent. That was nearly four percentage points under the average. However, by 1993, investor-owned hospitals were managing Medicare patients better than most. Their margins were still in the red, but only by one-half percent, and that was a full percentage point better than the industry average. In an early 1994 article in *Barron's*, legendary stock picker Peter Lynch, vice chairman of Fidelity Management and Research Corp., lauds the prospects of investor-owned chains like Columbia/HCA's to compete. "Well, 85 percent of the industry is nonprofit. And, the not-for-profits are nice folks to compete against," Lynch said.

That's true except for one thing. If times get hard, not-for-profits may be able to outlast investor-owned hospitals. When things get tight, the not-for-profit is more likely to hang in there; the for-profit will be sold, closed, or go through a revolving door of administrators. However, that's a worst case scenario—not the type of thinking that goes on at the negotiating table. Especially if those doing the negotiating are former not-for-profit executives themselves.

That was the case at American Medical International, which was purchased this year by National Medical Enterprises. After Dallas-based AMI hired former not-for-profit executive Robert O'Leary in 1991, O'Leary set off to buy not-for-profit hospitals.

O'Leary, a former St. Joseph Health System president and CEO, was recruited by AMI when he was president and CEO of Voluntary Hospitals of America. The bait was $1 million in salary, a $400,000 signing bonus, and a loaded stock option plan. VHA is the nation's largest alliance of not-for-profit hospitals, a base that gave O'Leary plenty of contacts to pursue. Interestingly, he was unable to capitalize on them. O'Leary bought only two not-for-profit hospitals during his tenure at AMI, neither of which had been VHA members.

The largest deal of the two was the $92 million purchase of St. Francis Hospital in Memphis, which became AMI's largest hospital. John Casey, AMI's chief operating officer, had formerly run Memphis' second largest hospital, Methodist Health System, and his contacts in Memphis proved useful in the St. Francis deal. To show what a small world the hospital industry is, Casey was the 39-year-old president and CEO of PSL Healthcare Corp. when that Denver hospital system was sold to AMI for $178 million in December 1984. At the time, the transaction was the largest purchase of a not-for-profit hospital by an investor-owned chain.

PSL owned three Denver-area hospitals, including its flagship 483-bed Presbyterian-St. Luke's Hospital. Casey coordinated that deal, then left before it closed to take the top post at Methodist in Memphis.

Fast forward to 1994. Casey is now working for AMI, and he hears that St. Francis is being wooed by his old employer, Methodist. AMI swoops in and cinches the deal. "The talk around town was Methodist would get the hospital and the (St. Francis) foundation would get a thank-you note, or AMI would get the hospital and the foundation would get a check," said William Billingsley, executive vice president of Eastwood Medical Center, another investor-owned hospital in Memphis. The Roman Catholic hospital's board took the check. Even though Methodist was offering a partnership to St. Francis, the board "saw that as losing to us," noted Maurice Elliott, Methodist's president. Competitive juices die hard. AMI paid St. Francis $92 million for the hospital. Putting the money into a community foundation made the board feel like heroes. Almost immediately, AMI started paring staff and closing patient units in the 16-floor hospitals. Jake Henry, the hospital's newly appointed CEO—and another former St. Joseph executive—told the *Memphis Healthcare News*, "Our investors do expect a return on their investment, and we have not been shy about saying that."

A CATHOLIC SYSTEM TURNS FOR-PROFIT

In this business, when you've seen one deal, you've seen one deal. Although experts abound in this business, every deal is different. Timing and people—they're never the same. Here are a few examples.

In 1993, Healthtrust executives, who had been busy turning around dozens of former HCA hospitals, decided to gear up into the acquisition mode. Healthtrust's CEO R. Clayton McWhorter was back in the saddle, having turned operations over to COO Hud Connery earlier in the year while McWhorter weighed a bid for the Tennessee governorship. In June, McWhorter scrapped the idea of running for governor, and Healthtrust became a buyer like many of its cohorts.

The Congregation of the Sisters of Holy Cross, Notre Dame, Indiana, decided to take bids for its Utah hospitals: 200-bed Holy Cross Hospital in Salt Lake City, 39-bed Holy Cross Jordan Valley Hospital in West Jordan, and 239-bed St. Benedict's Hospital in Ogden. These hospitals were perfect for Healthtrust, which had six hospitals in Utah, four of which were in the Salt Lake area. None of the Healthtrust facilities were big enough to provide tertiary care, however.

Healthtrust was one of the early entrants on the network bandwagon and McWhorter, Connnery, and their development executives really wanted Holy Cross Hospital for a hub in downtown Salt Lake City. They had a motivated seller, a Catholic system that had seen profits plummet the year before to a thin $648,000 on revenues of $89 million.

"Healthtrust was selected in part because of its facilities along the Wasatch Front and its existing partnership with us as well as its commitment to compassionate, high-quality, and cost-effective care," said Sister Patricia Vandenberg, the system's CEO, announcing the deal on October 1, 1993. Healthtrust also was selected because it had the high bid: $140 million. (That amount later was discounted to $125 million, however, after Healthtrust inspected the assets and saw some capital improvements were needed.)

The acquisition was a major coup for Healthtrust, an arrangement that would give the company ownership of 7 of the region's 23 acute-care hospitals or a 30 percent share of Wasatch Front market, which had a little over 1 million residents.

At first, everyone was smiling, but the smiles would soon end and turmoil ensue. First, contributors (both Catholic and non-Catholic) who had supported Holy Cross through the years began calling the office of the Most Rev. William K. Weigand, bishop of the Diocese of Salt Lake City with questions such as, How could the Catholic church sell this hospital to a for-profit chain?

Weigand had given tacit approval to the deal after being assured by the Sisters that they'd tried to sell the hospitals to another Catholic system. Keeping the hospitals under Catholic control was an option that he felt should be exhausted before the Sisters even considered selling to an outsider. That was especially true since the outsider was Healthtrust, an investor-owned company.

Officials from the Sisters' organization told Weigand they'd exhausted the options, but apparently Weigand was somewhat skeptical. He started making his own calls. One potential buyer was the Sisters of Charity of the Incarnate Word Health System (Incarnate Word), an 11-hospital system based in Houston. The Sisters of Charity didn't own a hospital in Salt Lake City but was investing $15 million there in long-term-care projects. Incarnate Word was building independent and assisted-living facilities, adult day care, and other services for the elderly in Salt Lake City, so it seemed logical the system might want a few hospitals, too.

The bishop called Houston and found out that Incarnate Word had never been contacted by Holy Cross. That was just the ammunition Weigand needed. He called Holy Cross officials, who in turn sheepishly phoned Healthtrust executives with the request, "Could we get your permission to talk to Incarnate Word?" "No!" came the adamant reply of Healthtrust executives. Not only no, but Healthtrust executives warned that such an act could be considered tortuous interference, a legal red flag. In other words, trying to break up a legal contract was going to carry legal implications.

Weigand didn't accept that response. He hopped on a plane to Rome to urge the Pope of the Catholic Church not to approve the sale. Whenever the Catholic church sells assets, it must get papal approval, a special permission known as an *indult*. Weigand got a 30-day suspension in the indult, then flew back to Washington to meet with a group of bishops, where he railed about the sale of the Catholic hospital to the "for-profiteers" from Nashville.

Healthtrust officials found themselves in a difficult position. They wanted the hospital, but responding to the bishop's declarations wouldn't exactly be a public relations dream. All that considered, Healthtrust convened a meeting of everyone involved in Nashville. Weigand was there and "immediately start[ed] talking about how he [was] going to make our lives miserable," said one Healthtrust source. Instead, Healthtrust attorneys informed him of the legalities of the Holy Cross contract and that breaking that contract now would make it appear that the Catholic church was not negotiating in good faith—an interesting legal and ethical consequence. The Most Rev. William K. Weigand backed down. He went back to Salt Lake. He said he would no longer stand in the way of the sale. He was subsequently transferred to Sacramento, California, although his transfer wasn't necessarily related to the Holy Cross sale. The arrangement was signed on December 6, seemingly marking an end to Healthtrust's problems in Salt Lake. But it was a short-lived hiatus.

As with any deal involving a competitive market, Healthtrust filed the required paperwork to receive federal antitrust clearance of the deal. If the Federal Trade Commission was going to stand in the way, it had 30 days to notify Healthtrust. For 29 days, officials heard nothing. Two hours before the notification period expired, the FTC filed a "second request."

That meant trouble. The FTC wanted more information so it could seriously consider the antitrust implications of the deal. A second request almost always meant the FTC would break up the deal; and even if the agency didn't, it would cost Healthtrust millions in attorneys' fees and added delay. Before the transaction was finally completed, Healthtrust would spend more than $1 million in attorneys' fees, trying to get the deal done, arguing unsuccessfully that the deal was pro- not anti-competitive.

Intermountain Healthcare (IHC), a 22-hospital health system with a dominant market share in Salt Lake City, was the anticompetitive one, Healthtrust executives argued. Merging Holy Cross' hospitals with Healthtrust facilities would create a strong competitor to the giant IHC. The feds were not convinced. Ten months after the original parties had agreed to the arrangement, the transaction was completed, but Healthtrust couldn't keep the downtown hospital. As part of the federal ruling, Healthtrust had to sell the most desired facility and did so less than six month later to Champion Healthcare Corporation, out of Houston.

Some ill feelings remained in Salt Lake City. Shortly after the sale, 12 lay members of the Holy Cross Health System's Utah board stepped down over a dispute on how the sale proceeds would be distributed. Monsignor M. Francis Mannion, rector of the Cathedral of the Madeleine in Salt Lake, was quoted by the Associated Press as saying the deal generated both disappointment and mistrust, adding that, "When the history of the sale of Holy Cross Hospital is finally written, 1994 will not be a shining moment."

Interestingly, Utah emerged as one of the few sites where the proposed merger between Healthtrust and Columbia/HCA ran

into snags. Again the issue was antitrust, and once again, the behemoth resolved the government's concern by divesting three of its
several hospitals in the state.

MIXING MISSION AND MONEY

Just because investor-owned chains are taking over religious hospitals doesn't mean they must snub the spiritual aspect of the
business. Some do, but one chain— Health Management Associates—has not. HMA is the only hospital chain to display the fish—
the Christian symbol for followers of Jesus—in its company logo.
The company's longtime chief financial officer, Kelly Curry, was so
committed that he quit in 1994 to be a missionary in Ireland. He
walked away from $2 million in unexercised stock options when
he did so.

Yet, for-profit healing is no more of an oxymoron than socially
responsible businesses, such as Ben & Jerry's Ice Cream or the Body
Shop.

Again, no profit, no mission, as the phrase goes. Indeed, in a
November 1994 research report by Robertson Stephens & Company,
a San Francisco investment bank, authors Sheryl Skolnick and Gian-
na Prime admitted to the conflict in talking about hospital profits.
Hospital profits grew 18 percent in 1992 and 12.4 percent in 1993.
"That is, one can infer that every additional marginal dollar spent
on hospital bills went straight to profits: not good for our social
consciences but great for our portfolios," the report commented.

Is it socially responsible to invest in companies that must answer
to a faceless group of shareholders? Is it socially responsible to
demand quarter after quarter of profit gains? Yet, some would
argue that it's not socially responsible to be wasteful either, and the
healthcare industry—both for-profit and not-for-profit—has been
wasteful indeed.

For example, in the same Robertson Stephen report, the authors
use the example of the Veterans Administration hospital system—
the largest hospital system in the country, with an annual budget
of $17 billion.

"Nonetheless, we note that Columbia/HCA operates a system
with a comparable number of beds and only 75 percent of the

revenue of the VA, yet it still turns a profit for its investors," the authors report. One might ask which is the more socially responsible system.

NME'S TAINT ON THE INDUSTRY

Still, return on investment—a dictum of investor-owned companies—can become a dubious master. It's 9 A.M. on June 27, 1994, in U.S. District Judge Kendall's court in the federal building, downtown Dallas.

The first case is a 19-year-old bank robber. He cries. He pleads guilty but says he's sorry. The judge, unmoved by the emotional display, sentences him and moves on. The second case is another bank robber. So is the third.

Next two are mail fraud cases and then another bank robber. Finally, it's the United States of America versus Pete Alexis. Amid these criminals, stands a former hospital administrator and regional vice president for National Medical Enterprises. As unlikely as it is to see a hospital manager here, it's even more unlikely to hear him plead guilty to paying between $20 million and $40 million in bribes to keep NME's psychiatric hospitals full in Texas. Judge Kendall asks Alexis if he paid doctors. "Yes," Alexis admits. Who else participated? Alexis explains that NME's psych divison had monthly meetings in Washington with the company's senior managers. "So, it was a companywide scam?" Kendall asks. "Yes, your honor," Alexis answers. Alexis and others will contend that NME's corporate bureaucracy instructed them how to perform the acts that are now threatening to put them in jail. Mark Jackson, a Kansas psychiatric hospital administrator, gets a three-year sentence while maintaining he was only doing what NME told him to do. Alexis, however, received probation—no jail time—because he was extremely helpful to the feds, who had hauled out dozens of boxes of patient records in a sting operation on NME headquarters. In an industry that speaks its own language, federal agents were overwhelmed with trying to figure out how to make indictments on the abundant information they had.

NME's psychiatric operations are an example of business principles gone awry. The entire system was bottom-line oriented, making every manager responsible for certain financial goals.

Obviously, that's admirable when making cars or flipping hamburgers. But, it takes on a new meaning, and new abuses, in the delicate art of treating mental illness. Regardless, the goals were set, and the underlying philosophy was to do what it took to meet them.

The things that NME employees would do to meet their bosses' expectations would become the subject of a wide-ranging government investigation. Later, NME would settle the case by agreeing to pay $379 million in fines and damages.

An atypical case? Yes. However, NME's excesses haunt the investor-owned industry. In some cases, it will be reason enough for tax-exempt hospitals to rebuff an offer from an investor-owned chain.

Chapter 7

To Align or Compete—The Crucial Considerations

Of course, the question of whether to align with, or compete against, Columbia or any of the proprietary systems is one that many providers have already faced. The key point is that in the not-too-distant future, many more will face the pivotal decision. Throughout the book, we have reviewed situations of hospitals that wrestled with that decision. Reviewing the history of the investor-owned systems as well as outlining their underlying philosophy and modus operandi should provide a better feel both for what to expect on the national basis and in the local market.

Of course, we can only speculate on the eventual outcome of all this frenetic activity by the for-profit systems (which we'll do in Chapter 8 when we present possible scenarios for the future). Nonetheless it is highly relevant for an organization considering its future direction to evaluate the proprietary systems based on their track record and their current approach. Such an exercise should (theoretically) help all those in the industry who deal with investor-owned systems to have a better conceptual understanding of the chains and perhaps provide some insight on future direction and performance. Arguably, while these taxpaying players control less than 20 percent of the market, right now they control over 80 percent of the momentum.

One thing is predictable. As the proprietary systems amalgamate and consolidate, they will become an even more formidable force—on the national level as well as the local markets in which they have a presence. If you don't believe that hypothesis, ask somebody in Florida how much time they spend thinking about Columbia's next move; it's probably a good share of the workday.

All this underscores the need for extensive analysis of each market and each organization's goals and objectives in light of the changing landscape in healthcare.

COMPELLING NEED FOR ALL ORGANIZATIONS TO ALIGN

Some hospital and physician leaders mistakenly believe they are isolated from the calculated market maneuvers of the taxpaying managers. This is a precarious assumption to make. Even rural markets are going to be affected by the actions of the investor-owned systems, because providers in rural markets will eventually need to become part of a larger system.

The accounting firm of Deloitte and Touche conducted a survey on administrators' attitudes toward alliances in 1994. This oft-referenced survey highlighted the belief (by the large segment of hospital executives questioned) that the majority of hospitals will need to be part of some kind of network within the next five years just to survive. A few of the salient findings that came from the survey are listed below:

- 71 percent of survey respondents belong to, or are developing, integrated delivery systems.
- 81 percent said their hospitals will not operate as stand-alone institutions within five years.
- 67 percent felt that it's essential for acute care hospitals to have some form of PHO.
- 53 percent of those surveyed were redesigning or reengineering their hospital.
- 48 percent were implementing outcomes measurement and management programs.

Clearly, the majority of healthcare leaders in the United States recognize the need to be part of a larger network or be affiliated with a comprehensive system. Such a sentiment ties back to the discussion of managed competition. We noted that as the purchasers of healthcare (ranging from managed care companies to employer coalitions) get more sophisticated and powerful, they will exert a greater demand for consolidation among providers—meaning large, geographically (as well as programmatically) diverse systems.

Consequently, the question will not be whether to align with a larger network, but rather which network to choose. Stated another way, the issue is not whether a facility should select a for-profit system or remain independent, but whether it should select a for-profit system over another system in the market. Eventually, most markets will be distilled down to two or three competing systems. In almost all of these markets, one of these networks will likely be an investor-owned network, more often than not Columbia/HCA.

MARKETS ARE BECOMING TWO-SYSTEM TOWNS

Such a division (between a for-profit network and a not-for-profit network) has already occurred in many markets, and the trend toward this bifurcation will accelerate in the next two to four years. In our estimation, by the end of 1998, there will very few large markets with more than three systems. Even many of the midsize markets will have consolidated to only two or three competing networks.

Therefore, as healthcare leaders approach the decision on alignment, we recommend weighing the benefits of the proprietary option against the other options available in each market. Hospital leaders can't assume they can ride out the tide of the *consolidation craze* that characterizes healthcare today. Everyone needs to choose a partner. The core question is which one will lead the delivery system into the next millennium in the best position possible.

THE NEED FOR ADVANCE PLANNING

A sense of urgency surrounding the alignment question should drive strategic planning efforts. Many hospital executives have not been prepared for this question (let alone the response) regarding alignment with a for-profit system. The healthcare industry is moving at such a rapid pace that delaying this particular facet of the planning process may result in hastily made and poorly executed decisions, with ensuing ill-planned initiatives, suboptimal at best, if not catastrophic.

Therefore, we suggest that leaders map out the scenarios now, consider the alternatives, and determine the appropriate course of action for the next two years. Easier said than done, right? Here are a few issues to consider before making a decision and outlining the strategic direction on stone tablets.

The first consideration is strictly survival based. In other words, which alignment option keeps the institution viable while producing value to the community? Given that the market will ultimately answer this query, let us suggest a few market measures to evaluate in making this decision.

FUNDAMENTAL OBJECTIVES OF INTEGRATION

We would propose that there are fundamentally two factors to consider in assessing the effectiveness of any integration model. Admittedly, this is gross oversimplification, but we've narrowed it down to a palatable pair:

1. Decreased costs.
2. Increased market leverage.

For any integration initiative to succeed, it *must* accomplish both these objectives. Otherwise the effort is little more than an expensive (and usually exhaustive) exercise in futility. Let's discuss each of these variables separately.

Decreased Costs

Not surprisingly, given the recent furor over escalating healthcare costs, purchasers of health services will devote their energies to reducing overall costs. Rightly so. The industry has long been characterized by cost shifting or *shifty costing*, depending on one's perspective. Too little attention has been given to the inordinate increases in health sector spending—especially as contrasted to other price increases in the U.S. economy. Understandably, the purchaser power brokers in today's market will focus on price first and everything else second.

Translation: Healthcare providers must go through somewhat of a modification of their mind-set. Historically, providers have competed on quality. No longer. Under the new world order, employers and the companies that represent them (such as managed care organizations or insurance entities) will select hospital and physician networks on the basis of the premiums offered not premium quality. Whether this new criteria is correct or corrupt has little relevance. It is the order of the day, and we'd better get used to it.

Managed Care and the Need for Covered Lives.   In 1994, many blue-chip healthcare institutions (the preeminent names atop the medical marquee) saw red ink (i.e. financial losses) for the first time—an indicator that even the crème de la crème are not insulated from the "discount shopping" approach. As testimonial to this, note the recent alignment of the major cancer centers in the country, uniting in an attempt to develop strength in numbers and leverage in negotiating.

So what does this pricing paradigm mean for providers? Fundamentally, it means that *the one with the lowest cost gets the covered lives, and the one with the most covered lives wins.* Importantly, we did not state the "one with the lowest price" gets the covered lives. That is because price is a short-term variable that can be manipulated based on market conditions and competitive reaction. *Short-term* is the operative phrase. You can only price low (for an extended amount of time) as long as your costs are low. As the adage goes, "If you are priced at or below your costs, it's difficult to make it up on volume."

So whatever alliance is considered—taxpaying or otherwise—that alliance should offer a configuration that provides the greatest opportunity for (long-term) low costs. This cost superiority can be achieved through a number of variables including the following:

- Reduced staff.
- Fewer product lines.

- More cost-effective services.
- Effective vertical integration—physicians motivated to, and educated on, keeping costs down.
- Reduced supply costs.
- Effective management information systems that offer cost-effective methods of delivery.
- Optimally efficient distribution of services, such as home care, skilled nursing, outpatient services, and so forth.

The for-profit chains, especially Columbia, like to tout the tremendous savings available through purchasing clout. This is not an incidental consideration, as supplies typically account for a sizable percentage of a hospital's budget.

What may mark a shift in philosophy from previous investor-owned systems to the investor-owned systems that are a force in today's market is that they have announced their intention to be a healthcare system, not just a hospital.

Delivery Models Are Moving Outside the Hospitals. The individuals responsible for healthcare, in the mid-1990s recognize that hospitals are limited in scope and strategy. The most efficient method of healthcare delivery is usually outside the hospital—far from the onerous overhead that is associated with traditional medical center operations. To the extent that integrated systems recognize the need to offer a continuum of healthcare and not just hospital care, they are more likely to effectively make the transition to increased capitated reimbursement and heavier penetration by the managed care organizations.

Profitability Requirements and the Impact on Current Market Prices. A very important element of the pricing/cost consideration is the margin requirement levied by the supporting organization. Predictably, the investor-owned systems are under greater pressure to realize higher margins. As was noted in the early chapters of the book, up until the past few years, not-for-profits actually outperformed the investor-owned hospitals on the bottom line. So even though not-for-profits have historically fared well in the profitability calculation, they are typically not under as intense pressure as the executives who manage publicly traded facilities. Of course, there are exceptions.

The turbulence of the past few years has provided several cases where CEOs of tax-exempt hospitals were removed from their positions due to the poor financial performance by their organization. (CEO turnover in hospitals was about 15 percent in 1994.) Nonetheless, in our observation the boards of not-for-profits are more lenient (and patient) in evaluating a CEO on his or her ability to meet budget in the short term than are the corporate chiefs who run the for-profits. This may be one reason why the investor-owned hospitals in many markets are higher priced—relative to their tax-exempt counterparts. Correspondingly, in a good many markets, the proprietary hospitals are *the* high-priced facility—forced to achieve their margin requirements through price increases as a surrogate for volume growth.

These margin requirements have placed some taxpaying hospitals in the precarious position of offering unusually high retail prices while attempting to maintain market parity for managed care. Significantly, as managed care proliferates in a market, the charge for commercial insurance or indemnity plans becomes nothing more than a hollow statistic. Eventually, the margins that once sustained the high-priced hospital dissipate, and the facility is faced with the prospect of stringent measures to reduce costs.

Many of the for-profit hospitals that operate in smaller or less sophisticated markets will face a rude awakening as their market assimilates purchasing cooperatives that are capable of (expeditiously) reducing prices. These employer coalitions bring the size and often the sophistication (having extrapolated the experience from other markets where they have sister facilities) to effect precipitous price reductions.

Obviously, such "out-of-sync" market pricing is not restricted to taxpaying facilities. We are familiar with a fair number of tax-exempt hospitals that are noticeably overpriced based on their competitors' charges. However, the high-priced leader board is more likely to be occupied by an investor-owned facility because they have been under the watchful eye of shareholders and the ensuing monthly and quarterly pressure to keep contribution margins up in a comparatively stagnant market. After all, how much real growth has there been in the healthcare industry in the past three years? Importantly, as capitation flourishes, we can expect to see operating income and other measures of profitability decline at a more accelerated pace than we've seen in the last few years.

System's Cost—the Crucial Factor. In making the crucial decision on alignment, healthcare leaders need to consider the cost position of both the publicly traded facilities and other competing systems. Pricing information for all the facilities is relatively easy to gather. Most hospitals' executives either have access to it or can obtain a detailed list on the "retail" prices for an institution. Many state hospital associations publish some form of pricing comparison, either DRG based or specified by major service and category.

Admittedly, published prices for commercial or indemnity business have little relevance in most markets. The critical variable is the facility's cost. This is slightly more difficult to obtain but not impossible. Much of the data—at least for aggregate measures—is available for a nominal charge through sources such as Medicare Cost Reports. Surprisingly, relatively few hospitals use these type of reports to assess their competitive position vis-à-vis their neighboring facilities. Even a few standard calculations or ratios can prove valuable in determining the cost position of potential allies or possible combatants.

For example, these macro ratios could prove helpful in evaluating the relative cost-competitive strength of potential partners:

1. Total costs per adjusted occupied bed.
2. Total costs per equivalent admission.
3. Total costs per equivalent patient day.
4. Labor costs per equivalent patient day.
5. Total costs per full-time equivalent (FTE).
6. Salary costs per FTE.

The first three ratios factor in outpatient activity, which is crucial in assessing the future competitive ability of the organization. Although it may be more difficult to obtain, a cost calculation without the outpatient component is woefully inadequate.

The latter three measures are focused on labor. For most hospitals, labor is the largest contributor to costs and is consequently the area that receives the most intense scrutiny after consolidation. If nothing else, a review of these above-listed calculations provides a preview of what an organization can expect to encounter following a merger with a proprietary system. If labor costs are way out of line with local standards, the hospital can anticipate some concentrated rightsizing following a merger or outright acquisition.

For those who are not able to obtain information related to these cost calculations through sources such as the Medicare Cost Reports, there are commercial references. One of the best sources for cost comparative data is listed below:

- *The Center for Healthcare Industry Performance Studies (CHIPS)*
  1550 Old Henderson Road, Suite 5277
  Columbus, OH 43220
  (800) 859-2447

CHIPS was founded by Dr. William Cleverly, a well-known expert in healthcare finance, and Dr. Roger Harvey. Both are affiliated with Ohio State University.

We strongly recommend an extensive review of each provider's cost position. As stated, if an organization selects the investor-owned alignment, it will have a preview of how much *organizational weight* it will have to lose following the marriage. If that same organization doesn't select the for-profit network or system as its partner, at least the managers will know what they're up against in terms of pricing in a competitive market.

Surprisingly, many hospitals do not take the time and effort to gauge the cost component when they're weighing the considerations for alignment. If cost is the lead driver on the healthcare highway, doesn't it make sense to assess the market cost position vis-à-vis the others before selecting a long-term partner? Obviously, Rick Scott and the Columbia/HCA executives are committed to being the low-cost provider in every market in which they operate. As mentioned in Chapter 4, this is the fulcrum on which the Columbia strategy pivots.

Consequently, cost should be a significant consideration in evaluating partners for the future.

Increased Leverage—Market Presence and Position

Historically, when a hospital measured its market share, it did so based on inpatient volume, outpatient visits, or a combination of the two. What is relevant in today's environment is what is carefully (yet necessarily) referred to as market leverage. The entire issue of market leverage has come to the fore because of the shift from quality to pricing as well as the shift in the power base of the players who now control healthcare.

In the past, big was better. Usually the 800-bed hospital was the 800-pound gorilla in the market. The large, tertiary hospital had the most physicians on its staff and offered the greatest array of services and expertise. However, in an environment of increasing payor savvy, risk-bearing necessity, and rising employer clout, the 800-bed hospital could end up the 8000-pound beached whale if it fails to effectively make the transition to the new order of healthcare. Research conducted by various healthcare providers in the process of developing networks shows that employees are not as interested in the location of a hospital as they are the location of their primary care doctor. While this may come as a blinding flash of the obvious to some, the hospital and physician leaders who conducted such research found it somewhat revelatory. As a consequence, one recently created network redirected its focus toward developing satellite primary care clinics.

In the past, the automatic response to network development would have been to put up another hospital or ambulatory surgery center within striking distance of the targeted population. Under the new order of healthcare, an employer interested in offering a comprehensive network to its employees is likely to be more interested in the availability of a workers' compensation program than services located on a hospital campus. Importantly, a statewide employer will be intrigued by a network of facilities and services that can be accessed by its employees anywhere in the area. Such a service is likely to be of far greater value than a complete array of services under one roof.

Variables to Consider in Assessing Market Leverage Possibilities. Each market is different. Consequently, the gauges required to assess each particular situation will vary. However, a few of the essential variables to consider are listed below:

- Managed care penetration.
- Number and strength of physician networks.
- Concentration of large employers and/or efforts at business coalitions.
- Percentage of Medicare and Medicaid population.
- Relevance of price competitiveness in gaining and maintaining contracts.

Let's dissect one of these crucial variables, and determine how each factors into the overall assessment of strategic positioning efforts.

Managed Care Penetration. Managed care is both friend and foe. On the one hand, the impact of managed care has been beneficial to realign the healthcare financial incentives in America. Who can argue with the concept of hospital leaders and physicians more concerned about keeping people away from the hospital (by keeping them healthy), than hoping the hospital is full? We have capitation to thank for that imminent shift in managerial mind-set.

Yet, managed care organizations have also had the effect of driving a (figurative) wedge between purchaser (employers) and providers (physicians and hospitals). In the process, HMOs and their managed care cousins (EPOs, PPOs) have made fortunes in the business of healthcare without treating the patient. Now hospital administrators and physicians are like disturbed wasps: angry and aggressive. (If you want to stir up the doctors in a hospital, cite the recent quarterly earnings of the local managed care organization.)

Admittedly, the managed care companies merely capitalized on what could be termed another golden opportunity, namely the unmet need for someone or something to monitor and control escalating healthcare costs. They have definitely achieved that, proving once and for all that capitation is the consummate mechanism for cost control in the healthcare industry. A study conducted by Foster and Higgins in early 1995 revealed that the rate of increase for healthcare costs in the United States had declined for the first time since Ben Franklin charged for prescription glasses. Or at least, that's how long it seems.

The point we want to make relates to the relevance of being a costcentric organization. Although this may be apparent to many in the industry, the impact of capitation will be to penalize over-head-laden facilities. Conversely, the organizations that are lean and mean will be the long-term victors.

In truth, hospitals and networks that trim their costs will be winners either way: whether there is capitation or whether traditional reimbursement is maintained. Able to offer the lowest price to managed care organizations, cost-focused health systems will be much more attractive in competitive contracting. Hospitals with lower actual costs will be better positioned to either accept a percent of premium from the managed care organization (in a collaborative arrangement) or offer direct contracting arrangements with large purchasing cooperatives or large self-insured companies.

Therefore, Columbia/HCA's approach to the managed care market—namely that it will not directly compete with HMOs (by assuming financial risk)—is a strategy that could be reversed in the future if the company so decided. For the present, Scott's expressed strategy to be the low-cost provider in each market is one that will serve the company well in either direct contracting or as a provider in managed care networks.

MANAGED CARE PROSPERITY MAY PROVE TO BE A LIABILITY

Interestingly, managed care companies are beginning to feel the backlash of their prosperity. In response to public (and purchaser) pressure, and in light of overall declines in the rate of medical inflation, HMOs have announced a rollback in premium increases for 1995. In early 1995, the California Public Employees Retirement System (CalPERS) pushed its managed care organizations to reduce their premiums (for the second straight year) in response to hefty reported earnings.

In our opinion, the public's consternation and concern over a $15 aspirin tablet is likely to shift to the stratospheric profit margins of managed care companies. Hospitals and physicians would be intuitively wise to stress such atypical prosperity in the healthcare field in light of public anxiety regarding the high cost of healthcare.

Susan Alt is an observer who has worked on the purchasing side of healthcare and now serves as a futurist/writer on healthcare strategy. Alt, who is executive editor of *Healthcare Strategic Management*, believes that the current growth and prosperity of managed care organizations has reached its zenith. She hypothesizes that large companies, either directly or through a vehicle such as a business coalition, will be attracted to the concept of "factory direct" purchasing or direct contracting with large provider networks. She feels that within three to five years many such purchasing cooperatives will have shifted significant volume to direct agreements with provider networks. She maintains that as the providers develop the expertise (either through acquisition or partnership) to handle capitation (claims and processing), the role of the financial intermediary will become redundant and market inefficient.

If Alt is correct (and she is not the only one predicting that such a shift will occur), the strategy of gearing up for accepting the insurance function will give provider networks a sizable advantage when large purchasers opt to deal directly with the provider community. So the strategy of being the low-cost provider, although unquestionably sound, may be insufficient. As stated earlier, the fundamental objectives of integration are to decrease costs and increase market leverage. Increased market leverage may be achieved through declining costs, but leverage is rapidly becoming a function of controlling the purchasing process. This control may be most effectively achieved by working directly with the ultimate buyer of services, which remains (and will remain) the employer or employer coalition.

SYSTEM PHILOSOPHY TOWARD VIRTUAL INTEGRATION IS KEY FACTOR IN ALIGNMENT DECISION

An important consideration in each provider's alignment decision then depends on the basic belief regarding the short-term position and long-term structure of the local market. If healthcare leaders feel that direct contracting arrangements may eventually supersede the traditional HMO mechanism, the tax-paying option may not be the best long-term strategy. For now, the investor-owned facilities do not seem poised or philosophically inclined to pursue a "virtual integration" strategy (i.e., incorporating the financing mechanism). Whether due to previous negative experiences with their own HMO debacles or the belief that low-cost positioning will provide sufficient market leverage, investor-owned systems do not appear as intent on pursuing direct contracting. On the other hand, some not-for-profit systems, such as Harris Methodist in Fort Worth, Texas, and other prominent leading-edge providers, have pursued a strategy of incorporating the financial function into the overall configuration of their network. In many of these networks, the financial component (HMO sector) has become the driver of the system.

In reality, however, very few not-for-profit systems or networks have sophisticated virtual integration strategies. Consequently, one of the most important factors to consider in the alignment decision is the fundamental faith in the provider community to develop its expertise in the underwriting function and either develop beneficial partnerships with insuring entities or develop that ability in-house.

Of course, there also remains the possibility of a mammoth organization such as Columbia bringing the financing expertise within its system in a rapid and thorough fashion by acquiring national HMO firms. Given the penchant for larger-scale acquisitions, the likelihood of Columbia achieving financial integration almost overnight is definitely within the realm of possibility.

As with all other decisions within the healthcare milieu, the optimal position relative to managed care strategy must be determined at the local level.

OTHER ISSUES TO CONSIDER IN SELECTING A PARTNER FOR STRATEGIC ALLIANCE

Physicians

We have discussed the philosophical approach that Columbia and the other investor-owned chains take toward the physician component. There is definitely an attraction to the Columbia/HCA option

for risk-averse doctors, but there is also the underlying consideration for some doctors who have a problem with proprietary
healthcare. Not all physicians are enticed by the prospect of equity
sharing or even the idea of increased remuneration. Many times,
physicians want involvement and control of the delivery process.
If the local networks, whether tax-exempt or taxpaying, do not offer
these options in the network, doctors may not be totally converted
to the integrated system.

Physicians are fiercely independent. The argument has been made
that younger doctors are not of the same mold, but there is still an
issue of autonomy with most doctors. Consequently, the ultimate
structure for the overall market network will need to align doctors'
incentives, both financially and philosophically. The experience of
the late 1980s and early 1990s (as related to physician compensation) teaches a valuable lesson in the need to gain the doctor's soul,
not just his or her pocketbook, in bringing him or her into the fold.
Fundamentally, if leaders of integrated networks focus only on
fiscal incentives, they will not engender the necessary cohesion with
the medical staff that will produce optimal competitive positioning
in the long run.

What's needed then is a thorough assessment of the medical staff
mind-set regarding the alternative networks in the community. One
of the most important lessons for all healthcare strategists to learn
(and live by) is that in the United States, physicians control the
process. Notwithstanding the influence of managed care and the
control it has gained, the doctor remains the fulcrum on which
healthcare delivery pivots. Aligning physicians with networks for
any market is a complex dynamic, of which individual financing
is an important, but not all-inclusive, component.

Community Sentiment

In many communities, the hospital is integral to the sociological
fabric of the area. The idea of corporate types from Wall Street
taking over the hospital may prove as foreign as tiramisu on the
menu of Joe's Bar and Grill.

Consequently, the attitude of community residents is an important factor to consider and gauge before choosing sides or selecting
a network option. The investor-owned hospitals have a reputation

(whether earned or not) for only treating *paying* patients. This is also likely to be an underlying concern of many community-based interest groups that will not relish the possibility of new ownership affiliation if it means that many local residents will go without care.

There is also the perception (and this one is widely held) that investor-owned facilities are higher priced and that their entry will precipitate higher healthcare costs for the community. Obviously, this is not always the case, but these perceptions are very real and often run deep. In considering opportunities for alignment, the potential partner will need to factor in all these issues.

For Columbia/HCA's part, they have proven to be masters at media control. Scott himself is a polished and articulate spokesman, and he has surrounded himself with a staff that understands the concerns of the various constituencies. The company's policy is to work with the local media—either through paid advertising or through the press—to effectively communicate the benefits of Columbia's involvement in the local community.

Not many people really understand the health delivery system in America. This is somewhat surprising given that healthcare now employs more people than any other private industry in the country. Still, if you ask Jill or Joe Public about the nature of for-profit hospitals vis-à-vis tax-exempt hospitals, they will likely give you a blank stare. In fact, in a survey conducted in the late 1980s, over 70 percent of the people questioned thought most of the hospitals in America were "for-profit" facilities. In reality, less than 20 percent of the hospitals were investor-owned.

Part of the media campaign by Richard Scott and the Columbia/HCA leaders is to elevate Americans' cognizance regarding the need for market reform, led by the industry leaders not the politicos. This is a sizable undertaking. Scott has made a strong case for the value of taxpaying institutions and the inherent economic inefficiency of tax-exempt organizations. Not surprisingly, this latter emphasis has not endeared him to the not-for-profit segment of the industry. In response, the VHA and other aligned organizations have recently mounted a campaign to educate Americans on the viability of tax-exempt hospitals, and the deep-seeded community contributions such organizations have historically provided.

There is an undergirding sentiment in the United States that healthcare should be available for all Americans. As concerned citizens, we are adamant in our belief that all our citizens should have access to medical care. Just don't ask us to fund it. This sentiment is not new in the 90s. Surveys conducted for decades have highlighted the core belief that healthcare is a right, not a "commodity." Consequently, there still exists a concern with and a misunderstanding of proprietary hospitals. Any leader of a healthcare organization should factor this fundamental issue into the equation in considering the eventual impact of alignment with a for-profit system.

Community response and support are perhaps the pivotal variables on which the alignment decision should be made. Fundamentally, most hospitals feel their reason for being is to provide health services to the community in which they are located. This, then, should be a lead factor in determining which alignment option is optimal.

Chapter 8

What Lies Ahead

Ideally, this would be the part of the book where we'd forecast the future of the healthcare delivery system in America. (Then we'd move on to our definitive recommendations for balancing the budget.)

In reality, this is the section of the text where we consolidate the thoughts and predictions of market sages and distill them into a few pages of varying perspectives. It is then up to you to take these varied viewpoints, coalesce the collective wisdom, and determine what path the industry will take. (Feel free to consult Nostradamus' diaries if you think that would help).

Fundamentally, there are two extreme possibilities for the future of healthcare (as it relates to the role of investor-owned systems). Continued growth or eventual dissolution.

SCENARIO 1: CONTINUED GROWTH

On one end of the possibility continuum is the likelihood that the current surge of activity by taxpaying organizations is not just a wave, but a tsunami; the aftermath of which will produce an entirely revised landscape of healthcare as we currently know it. Under this scenario, the for-profit companies will continue to grow and consolidate to the point where they represent one-third of all the hospitals in America.

This monumental presence will be accomplished through mergers of the largest firms followed by acquisitions of not-for-profit, unaffiliated hospitals. Following this scenario, the taxpaying megafirms (or firm) will grow to over 2,000 hospitals. Eventually, 1,000 of these facilities will be closed or redesigned for other services.

In the tax-exempt sector, and in the wake of this corporate colossus, over 1,000 not-for-profits will end up shutting down or being absorbed into larger networks, leaving a total of approximately 3,200 private hospitals in the country. In this dramatically reduced environment, where 1,000 of the nation's private hospitals are taxpaying entities, the for-profit sector will not only command over 30 percent of the total market, but a significant position in every large MSA in the country.

These hypothetical numbers (of consolidated and eliminated hospitals) are not that preposterous when one considers the potential impact of increasing levels of capitation and the concomitant need for dramatic downsizing in the overall system.

In its study, *Hospital Networking: Mergers, Acquisitions and Affiliations*, the Healthcare Advisory Board developed a scenario for the "post-modern era" wherein the market was characterized by the dramatic shifts noted below.

	1994	*Post-Modern Era*
HMO penetration	15%	70%
Capitation	6%	50%
Hospital Days/1,000	830	285
Hospital Beds in use	590,000	200,000
Hospitals	5,200	3,500

Interestingly, the Advisory Board followed this controversial forecast with empirical research that demonstrated how, historically, hospital closure has had little correlation to reduced demand. Figure 8–1 depicts the declining occupancy rates for American hospitals vis-à-vis the total number of hospitals in the United States.

Even more telling is the message in the accompanying bar charts (Figure 8–2), which describes the status of "financially distressed" hospitals five years after they were determined to be in trouble. As these numbers demonstrate, hospital closures do not occur readily— nor necessarily in response to market conditions.

Interestingly, as we have mentioned, one of the most important activities that Columbia and other taxpaying companies have introduced into the healthcare milieu is the demonstrated ability (and tendency) to close hospitals. Correspondingly, the post-modern scenario outlined by the Advisory Board is more likely to occur with continued activity by the investor-owned firms.

FIGURE 8–1
Problem of "Sticky" Supply

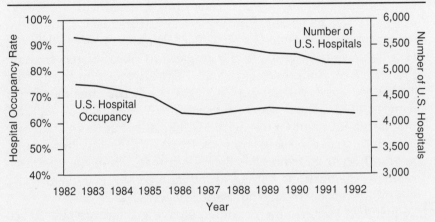

Excerpted from: Hospital Networking: The Advisory Board Company, 1994

Source: *AHA Hospital Statistics*, 93/94 Edition, 92/93 Edition, American Hospital Association, Chicago, Illinois

FIGURE 8–2
The MacArthur Axiom—"Old Hospitals Never Die"

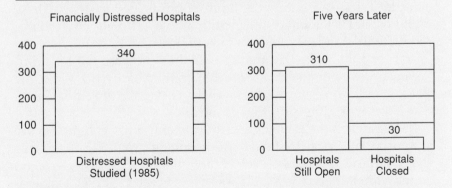

Study concluded that closure rates for distressed hospitals are comparable to those for the hospital industry as a whole

Excerpted from: Hospital Networking: The Advisory Board Company, 1994

Source: *Effects of Horizontal Consolidation on Hospital Markets*, American Hospital Association, Hospital Research and Education Trust, Chicago, Illinois

There are, of course, those who predict an even more dramatic impact on the tax-exempt hospitals in the country. One of these prognosticators is Paul Queally, a venture capitalist with the Sprout Group, which provided funding to Houston-based Champion Healthcare. According to Queally, "The religious orders will be out of the business in 10 years. It's no longer the Cabrini Sisters treating immigrants on the Lower East Side." Queally goes on to say that "healthcare has become a big business. As it becomes more of a business, the business people will win." We seriously doubt Cardinal Bernadin would agree with Mr. Queally, but there are many in the industry, especially those with ties to the investor-owned sector, who would echo Queally's sentiments about the business-oriented organizations having an advantage over the historically mission-driven hospitals and health systems.

Given this scenario then, where taxpaying titans are able to see their dream become a reality and are able to maintain margins and investor confidence, what is the probable fate of the two thousand remaining not-for-profit institutions several years and myriad market changes down the road?

No doubt these tax-exempt organizations will have to become more "business oriented" to counter the Wall Street wonders with which they compete in virtually every major market. This fine-tuning of business acumen has already occurred in many tax-exempt facilities—especially the large, sophisticated systems. These multihospital contenders offer comparable information systems, productivity standards, and obvious clinical quality. Some industry pundits would argue that there is still "fat" in these not-for-profit organizations, but based on research conducted by the VHA, the staffing ratios are comparable and the cost structure in line with many of the leading proprietary facilities.

In question is the issue of charity care and what volume of care is appropriate. Are the taxpaying hospitals providing their "fair share?" This is, of course, a calculation that must be considered on an individual market level; the issue that is relevant (yet problematic) is what constitutes a fair share for a taxpaying facility that is not receiving any subsidy from the federal or state government. As Rick Scott and others have vehemently argued, "Give the investor-owned hospitals the subsidies currently afforded the tax-exempt hospitals, and the nation (and individual markets) will see parity in charity." This is obviously an improbably reconciled catch-22, as few of the not-for-profits would be willing to abdicate their tax-subsidized assessment or their stewardship to care for the underserved and the uninsured.

The wild card in this deck of high-stakes healthcare poker is the future configuration of Medicaid and Medicare. The current Congress has its aim on the target of a balanced budget. As of this writing in 1995, Medicare and Medicaid appear to be two of the most promising silver bullets for hitting the bull's eye. The most probable mechanism for reducing costs in both of these budgetary behemoths is the same reimbursement structure that appears to be working for the private side of the healthcare ledger: capitation, under a managed care arrangement.

If a concerted push is given to capitate the federal programs for healthcare reimbursement, the type of competition we are seeing now will look like a gentle game of badminton compared to the hard-ball healthcare we could expect to see under a Medicare and Medicaid capitation system.

What this means for the "traditional" sector of healthcare delivery in the United States can be summarized as follows:

- The focus on cost will escalate—especially through the turn of the century.

- Community-based programs that offer relevance but not revenue will be reduced if not eliminated entirely.

- Consolidation and alignment will continue among the tax-exempt to counter the aggregation among the taxpaying systems.

- There will be pronounced bifurcation (between the two orientations) in individual markets, with physicians and other players in the healthcare arena choosing between the tax-exempt or taxpaying sectors.

- Providers on all sides will make an effort to deal directly with the end purchaser—large and medium-sized employers or business coalitions.

- Managed care organizations will initially offer a broad range of provider networks but will eventually be forced to align with one camp: taxpaying or tax-receiving.

Such is the scenario at the one end of the continuum which favors the for-profit mechanism, and continues their momentum.

EVENTUAL DISSOLUTION OF INVESTOR-OWNED HOSPITALS

At the other end of the possibility continuum, as related to the impact of the investor-owned sector, is a scenario where the tax-paying tidal wave is merely "déjà vu all over again" (to quote the inimitable Yogi Berra). In other words, the 90s are merely a remake of the surging 70s, with a few names changed to modernize this most recent episode. Predictably, in this version of *As Healthcare Turns*, the high-profile, high-flying years (1992 through 1996) are followed by the inevitable downturn in the financial markets and the subsequent dissolution of our contemporary conglomerates.

One industry pundit predicted, "These systems cannot continue to maintain their phenomenal growth. Once the burden falls to making the system operational, the true challenge will surface and the not-for-profits will have an advantage."

These comments echo the sentiment of many industry observers and experts, who wonder about Columbia's ability to forge a superior system out of a hodge-podge of clashing cultures and varying operational styles. As has been noted earlier in the book, the momentum can be maintained as long as the corporation's growth is being amassed through acquisitions and mergers on a large scale. Once the big fish are brought into the boat, however, can Columbia continue to propel itself on individual hospitals. These single acquisitions prove resource-intensive to assimilate, and offer minimal impact on overall revenues and profitability?

Once the large systems, from Columbia to OrNda, have to garner momentum from the operational efficiencies of their systems, will this be enough to hold the interest and intrigue of Wall Street investors and Main Street supporters?

The naysayers in the audience would argue that, as we pointed out in Chapter 1, the significant opportunities for meaningful margins have been seized. The big dollars in the system evaporated with the introduction of DRGs and, more recently, with the heightened awareness on the part of savvy purchasers regarding costs. To use analogous terms, healthcare no longer offers the large margins of jewelry stores. We're at grocery store levels in terms of profitability.

If this is true, and the efficiencies to be "squeezed out" of the delivery system are largely illusory, then indeed the investor-owned systems have a sizable challenge ahead of them. In the early years of the 1990s, the industry witnessed the reemergence of the taxpaying hospitals atop the profitability ladder. Prior to that (in the late 80s), the not-for-profits recorded higher margins than investor-owned facilities. However, even with the proprietary systems once again on top of the leader board, the margins are still not worthy of much excitement, nor are they comparable to the numbers posted by Humana, HCA, and others during the heyday of the 1970s and early 1980s.

Given the trend toward ratcheting down healthcare costs, the focus on purchaser leverage, and the Republican Congress' commitment to reducing the fiscal girth of the nation through Medicare and Medicaid cuts, the question becomes, Where will the cost-efficiencies be derived?

Another critical question raised by skeptics concerns the ability of the investor-owned chains to adapt to managed care. "The bulk of what they're billing for is extremely vulnerable," noted Kevin O'Donnell, a healthcare consultant in Lewisville, Texas. O'Donnell goes on to say, "I think one of their areas of expertise is going to have to be the ability to efficiently close hospitals."

Obviously, closing hospitals is not the only strategy necessary to compete in the managed care milieu, but consolidating services certainly is an essential part of the game plan. A recent study by Milliman and Robertson, the well-known actuarial firm out of Seattle, concluded that 59 percent of the time patients spend in the hospital is medically unnecessary. The trend is toward shorter stays and moving people to less costly facilities or structures for healthcare delivery, such as home health or skilled nursing units. The question then becomes whether the investor-owned systems, which have historically focused on hospitals and hospital hybrids, can effectively integrate these "health system extenders." Rick Scott has stated on numerous occasions that his intention is to become a health system not a hospital chain, and the acquisition of Medical Care America is certainly anecdotal testimony to that tenet. However, the integration battle is waged on a local scale; therefore, the corporate culture must funnel down to the individual market and effectively execute integration strategies that will position each area network optimally for managing under capitation.

MOST LIKELY SCENARIO

So of the two scenarios, which is most probable? As stated at the outset of the chapter, these represent the far ends of the scenario spectrum. If we had to place our money on which scenario is closer to reality, we would select the former forecast, wherein the investor-owned momentum is maintained and the taxpaying hospitals assume a greater degree of market presence and industry influence. Here's why.

First, Columbia has the unique opportunity of benefiting from the industry's pioneers and patriarchs. It is rather rare to see an industry recycle itself in less than 20 years, but that is what's happened with the investor-owned sector. Additionally, the patriarchs are still around—in an advisory capacity—to warn of and ward off the evil presence of the ghosts of mistakes past. This is a highly unusual dynamic for any industry and, as mentioned earlier, a tribute to the confidence and sense of historical perspective possessed by Columbia's captain, Rick Scott.

No one knows how long Clayton McWhorter and Thomas Frist, Jr., will stay around, actively involved in the managerial affairs of Columbia, but as the saying goes, "Start right, and you'll usually end right." As for the other chains, relatively new players like Barbokow at Tenet will no doubt look to Columbia for leadership and models, as Columbia has not only the momentum, but the market magnates in its camp.

Reason number two that favors the for-profit facilities is the metamorphosis of the market. Earlier, we raised the significant question of the ability of tax-paying hospitals to manage managed care. The prominence and dominance of HMOs, PPOs, and OWAs (other weird arrangements) may be more of a help than a hindrance to investor-owned systems, which clearly have a focus on the ledger.

Back in the halcyon years (the pre-DRG era), the prominent variable in the healthcare purchasing equation was quality. As noted earlier, many of the proprietary hospitals struggled to be considered on par with their tax-exempt counterparts. (Recall the famed foray by Humana in its attempt to rivet quality on its marquee with the artificial heart episode.) Now the mood has shifted and so has the decision-making criteria. Major payors and purchasers of health services, for the most part, assume a high level of quality and therefore make a beeline to the bottom line. Cost is king for the power brokers who are buying healthcare services. This group is characterized by managed care executives who play providers against each other in bringing down the costs, and business coalition managers who represent multiple employers with myriad employees.

In this new game of hardball healthcare where price is the only real ball in play, the for-profit mind-set may be a differential advantage over its counterpart and competitor. We would venture that the for-profits have demonstrated both greater acumen and heightened tenacity in consolidating services and closing hospitals. For one thing, there is not as much emotion in the decision, which tends to slow the process if not derail it entirely. The perception of taxpaying administrators as bottom-line oriented, emotionless executives who can cut costs, reduce staff, and eliminate services may not get them a leading role in *It's a Wonderful Life*, but it may provide an upper hand in negotiating managed care contracts.

Under a market structure that involves high levels of capitation, the low-cost provider will eventually be the victor. In many markets, the low-cost provider position is occupied by the proprietary facilities, which have been ratcheting costs down for a decade or more, trying to bolster eroding margins. Granted, there may not be that much more to squeeze out of this turnip, so the margins may never be that attractive, but on a market-by-market basis, the investor-supported facility will be in a better position to offer bargain-basement pricing.

This is especially relevant as we consider the monumental move by the federal government to push Medicaid and Medicare into managed care. Bruce Vladek, who heads up the Healthcare Financing Administration (HCFA), has been quite clear that he wants "favored nation pricing" for Medicare and that managed care for federally supported health claims will become a reality. All the more reason to be the low-cost provider in any market.

Yet another reason deals with the governance structure of individual boards—especially unaffiliated, not-for-profit hospitals. We have heard from more than a few board members that they chose the investor-owned option out of frustration and consternation. Many board members (especially of the hospitals mentioned above) sit on the governance council as a service to the community. Often, their experience in healthcare is limited to the monthly or quarterly meetings they attend as part of their board responsibility.

But healthcare has become too complex for the part-time participant. What we're hearing in the field is that some board members are overwhelmed by all the changes affecting the industry. They are uncomfortable and under-informed on significant issues such as managed care, strategic alliances, vertical integration, and a host of highly relevant, extremely complex facets of the changing landscape. Sometimes in frustration, or desperation, these board members reach for something or someone who seems to have a handle on the industry and seems to be ahead of the wave—such as Columbia or another investor-owned system.

Not that all (or even most) of the boards across the country are in this somewhat apoplectic state. Yet there seems to be mounting frustration in dealing with these monumental changes. Hence, the option to "just turn it over to Columbia and let them figure it out," may be selected by a larger number of individuals in the ensuing months and years.

Why not sell to a for-profit provider? Because of the high standards hospitals must maintain to be Medicare hospitals, few question whether quality will suffer at the hands of a for-profit owner. In fact, the recent headlines about quality in hospitals surfaced at not-for-profit institutions. Consider the recent high-profile cases at Tampa's University Community Hospital—where surgeons amputated the wrong leg—and at Dana-Farber Cancer Institute—where a highly regarded health writer was killed by a toxic overdose. How different those news stories might have read if the two hospitals were owned by Columbia or another investor-owned chain.

Arguably, investor-owned chains must be even more diligent ensuring quality patient care. Because they are so fiscally oriented, corporations can't afford to be caught up in a scandal on the quality of patient care. The bottom line is that boards who sell out to Columbia or Health Management Associates rarely question whether quality will suffer at their hospitals. It seems to be a moot issue. Given that quality becomes a moot issue, the major issue remaining is money. Specifically, who best manages the nation's economic resources that pay for our healthcare services? Does Columbia manage our healthcare dollar best or does the Catholic church or does the local county government? Or is it a combination? In the final analysis, the individual market will determine the most effective structure. In essence, it all boils down to strategy—and that is carried out on a local basis. The clout and capital of a major corporation or a sizable system certainly provides leverage, but each market is different, and every situation is unique. The investor-owned systems are currently on a roll that is unprecedented in this industry, and with few parallels in any field.

Only the market will determine whether this resurgence by the investor-owned systems is truly a revolution or merely a temporary uprising.

Index

About the Authors

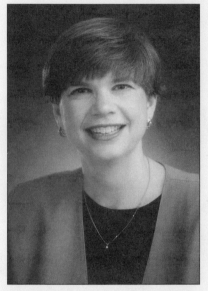

Sandy Lutz

SANDY LUTZ is Dallas' bureau chief for *Modern Healthcare,* a weekly business magazine that covers the hospital industry. Since joining the magazine in 1986, she has reported on investor-owned hospital chains as well as a wide range of healthcare finance topics, including reimbursement, stock and bond offerings, bankruptcies and restructurings. Ms. Lutz also anchors and edits a monthly satellite TV news magazine, *Health Reform Update.* Prior to joining *Modern Healthcare,* Ms. Lutz was managing editor of the *Memphis Business Journal,* and is a former reporter for the *Kansas City Times,* the *Lincoln (Neb.) Journal,* and the *Kansas City Kansan.* Mrs. Lutz is a native of Omaha, Nebraska, and received her bachelor's degree in journalism from the University of Nebraska–Lincoln. She lives in Arlington, Texas, with her husband and her two daughters, ages 6 and 11.

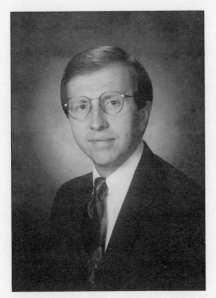

E. Preston Gee

E. PRESTON GEE is senior vice president, Marketing and Business Development for St. David's Health Care System in Austin, Texas. Gee has served in senior strategy positions for American Medical International in Missouri and Sacred Heart General Hospital in Oregon. Before entering the healthcare field, Gee spent several years in planning and market development with The Quaker Oats Company.

Gee is the author of several books, including *Thriving on Reform*, (Irwin, 1994), and has written numerous articles on industry trends. He is a frequent speaker on healthcare strategy for professional groups and industry leaders. He is a recent recipient of *Modern Healthcare Magazine's* "Up and Comers Award."

Gee received his B.S. and MBA degrees from Brigham Young University.

He and his wife, Janice, live in Austin with their six children.

Acknowledgments

We would like to acknowledge the contribution of the many individuals who have contributed time and ideas to this book. First, we want to thank the leaders of the organizations for which we work for their encouragement of this effort, Jack L. Campbell of St. David's Healthcare System and Clark Bell of *Modern Healthcare*.

We express our sincere gratitude to the many individuals who we interviewed for this book, and who offered valuable insight and perspective on the history and future of the for-profit sector. There are too many to list, but they are cited throughout the text.

A special thanks goes to those who reviewed the book and offered suggestions and encouragement, specifically Russell Coile, Jr., Ed Gordon, and John Runningen.

Finally, we are indebted to our spouses, Janice Gee and Larry Lutz for their patience and endurance while the book was being completed.

Other books of interest you you from Irwin Professional Publishing . . .

THRIVING ON REFORM
Meeting Tomorrow's Healthcare Challenges Today
E. Preston Gee
ISBN: 1-55738-618-8

NOT WHAT THE DOCTOR ORDERED
Reinventing Medical Care in America
Jeffrey C. Bauer
ISBN: 1-55738-620-X

STRATEGIC HEALTHCARE MANAGEMENT
Applying the Lessons of Today's Top Management Experts to the Business of Managed Care
Ira Studin
ISBN: 1-55738-631-5

HEALTHCARE MARKETING IN TRANSITION
Practical Answers to Pressing Questions
Terrence J. Rynne
ISBN: 1-55738-635-8